3 IN 1

BEST

FOOD RECIPES,

D.I.Y
SIMPLE IN-A-NUTSHELL WAYS

TO LOOSE WEIGHT FAST,

AND
EFFECTIVE NATURAL HEALTH REMEDIES BOOK.

Acknowledgment

TO YOU,
WHO PURCHASED THIS BOOK,
I love you

________   Clinton emscent

2

<u>Overview</u>

THIS BOOK HAS THREE
SECTIONS,

FOOD RECIPES ,Plus other

contents.

WEIGHT LOSS Including exercise

plans and meal plans

AND

NATURAL REMEDIES FOR

SOME SELECTED MAJOR

SICKNESS AND DISEASE

EACH SECTION HAS CHAPTERS
AND THEMES UNDER IT..

Each section is fully discussed
before heading to the other.

Please note: not all pictures on the
food recipes, represent the
food/recipes being discussed.

Appreciation

First of all,I want to say a BIG THANK YOU! to you for deeming it necessary to purchase this book with your hard earned money, thank you very much! And I really appreciate your support,and I trust that this book be all that you desire for it when you glanced at it…
I promise you won't regret your decision and choice today,as this has been a product of weeks if not

month (s)of writing and researchs
with personal references
I hope is worth every single cent of
yours

Thank you!!

Table of Content:

CHAPTER 5

SECTION ONE:

CHAPTER ONE:

60+ Simple fruit And Food Recipes:

MERMAID VEGGIE BOWL

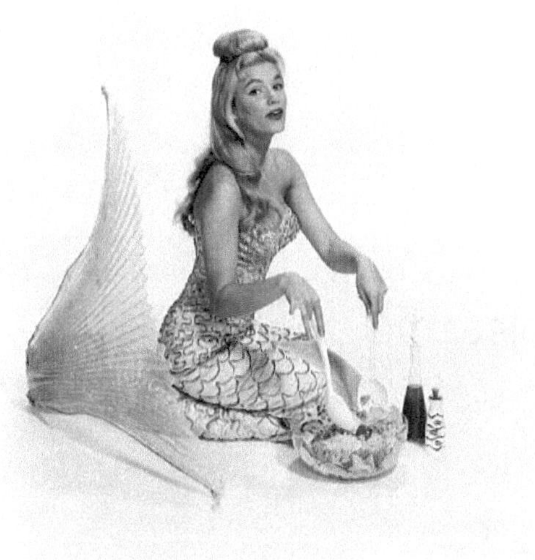

Cooking Time:
5-6 minutes

Servings:
2

Nutrient profile:
Dairy-free
Soy-free
Gluten-free

healthful Immunity
high Blood stress
excessive Fiber
Low fat

Egg unfastened
Bone health
healthy ageing
heart wholesome
excessive Calcium
Low-Calorie
Low Sodium
Vegetarian

Ingredients;
2 frozen bananas, peeled
2 kiwis, peeled
1 cup clean pineapple chunks
1 cup unsweetened almond
milk
2 teaspoons blue spirulina

powder

½ cup clean blueberries

½ small Fuji apple, thinly
sliced and cut into 1-inch
flower shapes

Fresh spinach leave(if desired)

Instructions:

Mix your bananas,and kiwis,
pineapple, almond milk and
spirulina in a blender,blend
excessively till it is smooth, about 2
minutes.

Divide the smoothie among 2
bowls. pinnacle with blueberries
and apples,add cucumber, and
spinach.

Nutrition information:
Serving size: 1 1/2 Cups
in line with Serving:

251 calories;
2.5 g general fats;
zero.three g saturated
fat; 116 mg sodium.
847 mg potassium;
59.5
g carbohydrates;
eight.7 g fiber;
36 g sugar; 4.eight g
protein; 488 IU nutrition

WATERMELON RADISH SALAD:

As said earlier,there isn't any Recipe you can't make out yourself, there are so many wholesome sweet Recipes for watermelon radishes,all you have to do is"think" it out,plan and execute your plan.

However it goes with different fruits and vegetables if desired,all together, you can combine with cabbage, cucumber, sesame, broccoli, spinach and or even mushroom! Yes really!

The watermelon radish offers the body a nice sweet nutrient and refreshment, which we shall talk about here…

Time:
5 mins

Servings:
2-3(varies)

Nutrient profile:
radish offers a great source of fiber, vitamin C, Calcium, potassium,
protein, carbohydrate and other nutrients, when consumed raw,the nutrients are in high quantity
Vegetarian
Low calorie
Low fat

Vitamins supplied
Perfect for your skin and health

Ingredients:
4-5 watermelon radishes
2 fresh cucumbers
1 1/2 cups microgreens
½ teaspoon peppercorns, slightly
crushed
1 peeled clove garlic
Fresh tomatoes
Spinach leave

Cooking instruction:
You can use a mandoline or any
slicer good to slice the watermelon
radish and cucumber,slice the
tomatoes equally "equally" haha if
you can! Of course you can! ,Now

place it all together in your plate or "ready-to-devour bowl", sprinkle a little salt,and add it all together,now see those micro Greens? Consider it as your decoration,and you will love the taste and the crispy light bite!

…. There's also an alternative method for this recipe...you can also boil some of the ingredients,simmer for some minutes and add a little water and vinegar,Incase you don't like eating raw tomatoes,you can cook it lightly…
Go ahead and make your own recipe from this,as you please! Yes you can!

Nutritional information:

Calories: 75.4kcal,
Protein: 0.7g,4.8g,
Carbohydrate:4.8g,
FAT: 6.1g,
Sodium: 520.5mg,
Sugar: 2g
Fiber active:1.4g.

SHAVED AVOCADO EGG TOAST:

Your perfect all season recipe! I know many people don't really like avocado ,that's okay,is normal not to love avocados! But with egg? Even with roasted would you still not want a bite? One bite fills your mouth,down to your gut to the main stomach chamber before going to the transformer haha but seriously this is one of the good solid foods around,you agree? Avocado has this speciality in it that makes you keep eating it,so soft and heavenly….for me I love avocado and I take it out with any Recipe that comes my way including, avocado and porridge beans,have you heard of it? Well ,if you haven't chill Emscent got you covered,I will share all the heavenly great soft recipes with avocados,one of my favourite foods haha yummy yum….

Ingredients:

3 hard boiled eggs preferably cold.
2 slices bread toasted
1 avocado
1/8 teaspoon red pepper,add
salt and pepper to taste...
1 radish thinly sliced
1 tablespoon chopped chives
lemon wedges for serving

Cooking instruction:

  Heat the saucepan over medium heat ,and once it starts to simmer, let it simmer for at least 1 minute!,allow them to cool off for at least 30 minutes,

Toast the bread lightly. Mash the avocado and add any additional seasonings you prefer (balsamic vinegar, nutritional yeast, lemon/lime juice, etc..).
Spread the mashed avocado on the toasted bread. Thinly slice the radish and use a grater to grate the hard boiled eggs. Add the radish and egg to the toast and add salt and pepper to taste! You can serve with lemon or a cold juice!

FRUIT MIX YOGHURT CREAM:

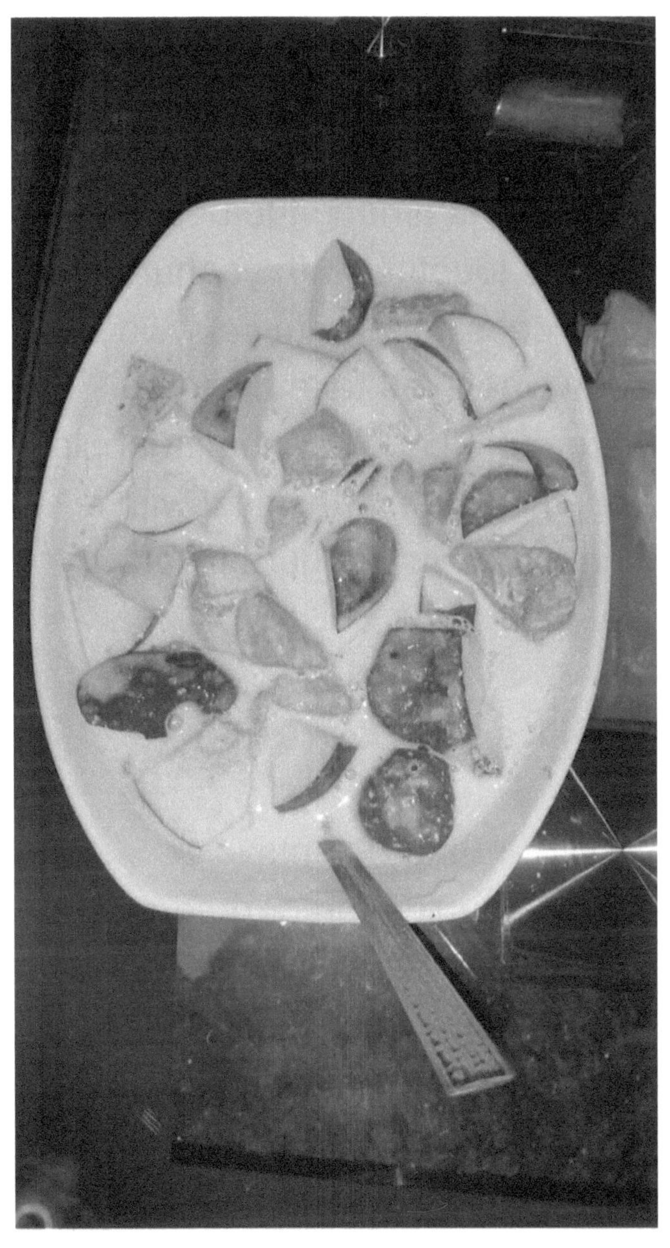

Well what else can I say? Your eyes have seen it all! …
With its mild and satisfying taste,this is among the best fruit recipes together with yoghurt mmm ,how does it feel with your whole body when you take a bite of watermelon,apple, and pineapple? Imagine accompanying it with a whole creamy yoghurt! If you haven't tried it…

Servings:
 2

Ingredients:
3 Fresh apples red or green!
½ cut watermelon from the whole body (you can use it all!)
½ pineapple from a whole fruit (depending on the quantity you want to make,you can put it all)

Yoghurt milk , you can make one or buy

      Direction:

  Get a clean bowl,wash your fruits,slice it all together to your desired sizes and shape
Put it all in one bowl
  And add your yoghurt milk!(or condensed milk) As simple as that!
Add some ice cubes in it yuuuppp!!!
  Ready to serve!

    Nutritional information:
High in vitamins... vitamins A,C,B
B12 etc
Contains potassium and magnesium
Good source of Calcium

Low carb
Saturated fat -lil
+small quantity of minerals from
Fruit

AVOCADO-PASTE WITH ORANGE AND VEGGIE:

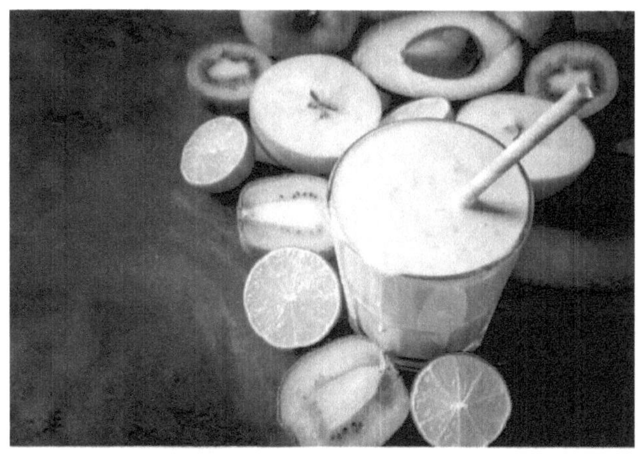

Ok you probably had never come across this avocado mixed fruit recipe,and like I said, avocado is like a goddess with so many spell casts (that's if goddesses use spell casts) ok that sounds like a nice joke,but avocado is also used like a butter,it fills up the stomach even enough for a whole day! Depending on the quantity taken

Avocado has a variety of vitamins and minerals it supplies, is a very good source of fat and oil,it's oil is great for our body …

Ingredients:
4 avocado pears
1 Sweet ripped orange
2-3 bananas
½ tablespoon of sugar
½ tablespoon of salt
A little cabbage
and any of your preferred veggie leave.

Directions:
First of all get two bowls or one plate and a bowl…
Peel off 2 avocados and squash,or blend it till it gets to a

butter form,or preferably a blender,till smooth…

Do the above with the banana,take two Bananas…

Now,make a sugar-salt Syrup (this is optional) with a very small amount of water and squeeze the orange juice into it,pour it together into the paste bowl and mix it all very well..

Chop your cabbage and spray it all over the pasta (this is optional)

Now the paste is done! Still have some Banana and avocado left right?.

Slice the avocado into desired sizes and shape,slice the banana aslo and put it all together,now you can add any of your veggie leaves….

Top with almonds or peanut

Now you have a bowl of
avocado-banana orange mixed
syrup bowl and a plate of sliced
avocado and Banana and your
favourite veggie leave!!!

Eat with a spoon for the bowl,and a
fork for the plate haha
Whoaaa! Enjoy!

   Note: you can also try out your
own recipe from this..Yes You Can!

TOASTED CAKE:

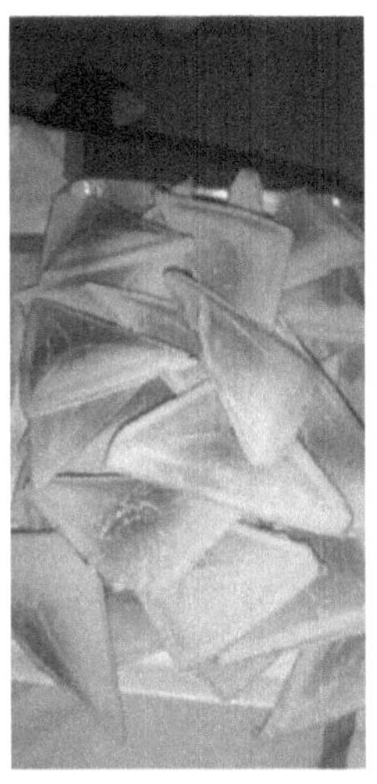

How to make toasted cake(without oven cake)
call it toasted cake.

So simple to make and you don't need to stress yourself using the oven whenever you want to have some cake ,it isn't much so let's rush through it…

   Good for the evening or even
breakfast.

Ingredients:
Butter
Sugar
Eggs
Milk
Floor
Pinch of salt
Baking powder

Direction:
So first of all have your normal
cake dough made,but let this
mixture be thicker than cake
Apply butter on both sides of the
toaster
Add 2 teaspoon on each of the
plates and have it closed.. Cook till

you get your desired brown or light brown color.

Give it a trial: this is making small cakes without using an oven…

Note: Do not attempt to close the toaster for too long, open it atleast after 10 seconds and close , but don't hork the pin until it turns brown

Served with juice or any drink…

TOTI WRAP:

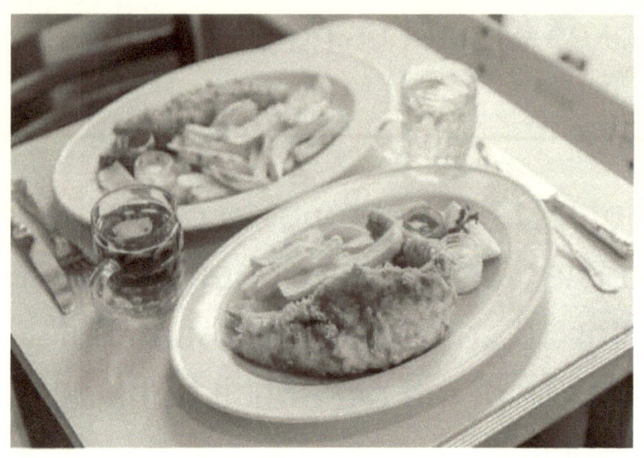

How to make a roti-wrap
Make a Tori wrap that can be
eating at any time of the day…

Servings :
5

Ingredients:

3 Cups of flour

4 tablespoons of Groundnut oil

½ -1 teaspoon of salt

270ml of boiling water

1 potato

1 tomato

1-2 onion

½ green paper

½ lettuce

Sausages

Mayonnaise

Cooking instruction:

Add dry ingredients together, mix
well with a ladder preferably, and
add water..
Let it blend Good,
Sprinkle some amount of floor on a
clean surface,after which,pour your
dough into the floured surface, put
the mixture, roll for about 5-7

minutes.. Once the dough is smooth, heat the pan, cut your dough in 6 equal parts, and roll it out until paper thin.. Place in a hot pan turning it other way around every 40 seconds
You Take 1 potato to fry,
1 tomato and cut it into strips
1 onion and cut into circles
Half green pepper cut into strips
Half lettuce
Sausages cut it into small pieces
Mayonnaise and any sauce of your choice

Nutritional information:
Calcium
Carbohydrate
Low carb
Minerals and vitamins supplied
Protein

Magnesium

FRIED SWEET POTATO TOSTADAS WITH CABBAGE AND SPINACH:

Nutritional Information:

Calories 148
Total Fat 8 g12%
Polyunsaturated fat 0.3 g
Monounsaturated fat 1.6 g
Cholesterol 33 mg 9%
Sodium 387 mg 17%
Potassium 250g mg10%
Total Carbohydrate 14g
Protein 10g 15%
Vitamin A 12%
Vitamin C 4%

Vitamin B-6 7%
Iron 8%
Cobalamin 8%
Magnesium 7%
Calcium 10%

Ingredients:

Corn oil
12 corn tortilla
Salt
3 ½ cups of refried beans, homemade or from 2 15-ounce cans
Cabbage chopped
Spinach chopped to your taste,
Potatoes
lettuce, sliced thin with vinegar no oil and salt
3 medium tomatoes, chopped

2 avocados, chopped peeled and
pitted, or guacamole
8 oz grated Monterey Jack,
Cheddar,cotija cheese(if need be)
One handful chopped cilantro
1 cup of salsa, or 1/2 cup sliced
pickled jalapeno

Cooking Instruction:

Warm the refried beans: Warm the refried beans in a frying pan on medium warmness, until warm. If you are using canned beans, drain them, then add them to the pan with a bit of water, mash them as they heat.

For extra taste for the beans you can stir in a tablespoon of bacon fat to them and,a huge slice of cheddar cheese.

Keep the beans on warm at the same time as you put together the tortillas, adding water to them as necessary to maintain a creamy consistency.

After that,   Dry the tortillas in oven: To assist the tortillas fry up better, dry them in the oven by means of laying them out on an oven rack and cooking them at 250°F for 10 mins

Pour sufficient oil into a frying pan so that you have a quarter inch layer of oil. Heat the oil on medium excessive warmth till sizzling hot, One at a time, fry the tortillas in the oil. Bubbles need to form within the

tortilla right now as you positioned
the tortilla within the oil, otherwise
the oil is not hot enough.
Fry till golden brown on both sides,
cooking about 30 seconds to a
minute according to the side. Use
spatula to push the tortilla down
within the oil, and to turn and lift the
tortilla out of the pan, draining the
excess oil as you do so,Get your
potatoes, depending on the
quantity you want to make,
Fry them lightly and drain oil,keep it
on a different pan or same plate
with your tortilla,add your chopped
cabbage and spinach leave spray it
on top

Add more oil to the pan as needed, taking care that the oil heats sufficiently earlier than including a tortilla to the pan.
Servings:
toppings in separate bowls, with a bigger serving dish for the beans.
Bring out the tostada shells in batches, preserving those unused warm inside the oven.
To prepare a tostada, unfold a big spoonful of mashed beans over a tostada shell. Sprinkle on cheese and different toppings sliced lettuce, avocados,and your fried potatoes on different pan
Enjoy with friends and family! With a chilled Drink!
Stay groovy!!

Coco choco:

Ever tried chocolate and coconut shake? I call it Coco choco,it can be served with bread, cassava fries or even any shake ,and can be enjoyed alone,it isn't hard to make ,as long as you have a reach to coconut,and   not   just   any coconut,but the tender ones,that their fruit is soft and unmatured

Ingredients:
1 Tender coconut
Powdered chocolate,or in any other form that pleases you..
Groundnut
Avocado or carrot

(Like I said,you can try any Recipe of your own! You just have to think it to live!,with reference to the ones you already know,....Come on it ain't going to be a crime if you get a little crazy in the kitchen..is it? Haha but be careful Because I won't be there….but of course I hope you understand what i am trying to say..BE CREATIVE! ….Yes You Can!!

Direction:
Let the coconut be an already peeled off bark one,cut it open like

a cup, just at the top please,you
can either drink half of the juice in it
or leave it all,(I leave it all) add use
a spoon,a ladle ,or a poacher ..if
there's any..just scrape the soft
fruit in it,you can either pour it out
unto a bowl or leave it at the
coconut cup(haha),let the fruit be
smashed or worked into being
creamy or close to a
semi-liquid,add your chocolate and
mix very well,

I prefer avocado if I'm going to eat
it with bread! But is your choice to
either use avocado or carrot and/or

altogether? Because it will make a great taste and savour on! The avocado alone should be if you want it all to be soft with no crisp ,just as the carrot will…

mix it all together,it should turn to a semi-dough or semi liquid ,but if you're eating with bread it should be sticky enough to hold on to the Bread or well ..just as you like it! Try it! You can also make it into honey-like and served chilled…...You Can try this with milk if you're a lover of milk..

CURRIED MANGO SOUP WITH Tomatoes:

Change your style of stew and soup with this fruit recipe,with unripe Mango,can be served with rice

ingredients:

5 unripe Mango
fresh pepper
4 fresh tomatoes blended
2 Onions
Teaspoon of salt
 maggi(season)
Pure oil (Groundnut or olive)
 Fresh fish
Curry

Cooking Instruction:

Wash the mango fruits, pill off the
back then slice it from the seed one
by one then cut them into your
desired shape and size
Cut onions
Have your fish or meat simmered
with spice preferably Curry and
onions

 add groundnut oil to your cooking
pot,
Add Onion fry for 5sec
Add ur paste
maggi and salt to taste,Pour in the
fish and it's water,add a few cup of
water,
Allow to boil for 10min

Lastly add the sliced mango leave it for 10min

Served with Rice ,or your preferred meal..

Good source of protein
Vitamin B12
Magnesium

HONEY MUSTARD SAUCE AND DRESSING:

ingredients

½ cup plain Greek yogurt (you can use a low fat dairy milk)

⅓ cup extra-virgin olive oil

¼ cup Dijon mustard

 4 tablespoons honey, to taste

2 ½ tablespoons of lemon juice

2 tablespoons apple cider vinegar

1 clove garlic, pressed or minced

 A pinch of fine sea salt to taste

10 twists of freshly ground black pepper

Any of your favourite vegetable leave

Instruction:

In a 2-cup liquid measuring cup or bowl, mix all of the ingredients as listed. Whisk until blended. Taste, and season with additional pepper if necessary.
This dressing is intentionally bold, but if it tastes too tart for your liking, whisk in another tablespoon of honey.

MASH-UP SAUCE RECIPE

Ingredients:

3 avocado pear
1 sizeable fresh tomato
 Almonds
Spinach (chopped)
2 tablespoons of lemon juice
Salt to taste
½ black pepper
Honey

mash up the avocadoes until they

are completely smooth, then begin

mixing in the tomatoes, onions, and

lime juice.

-firstly, Slice your tomatoes circular

Pour in the mashed avocado in a

bowl,add the lemon juice and mix

evenly.

Add a spoonful of honey to taste

,add black pepper

Add a pinch of salt ,

Boil/cook your spinach (not for long) have it chopped and pour into your bowl ,mix together with the content already in place.

Then add tomatoes and almonds for a crisp bite.

Serve with anything! Or just taken like that

CARB SMART SPICED PUMPKIN CHIPS:

Ingredients:(measure and add to your taste and desired quantity)

Blanched carrots
Carb smart beef
Black pepper
Chillies
Spinach
Pumpkin chips
Baby marrow
Carb smart braai spice
Cream

Cooking instruction:

To get your pumpkin chips,follow this method:

Preheat the oven to 220°F. Line 2 baking sheets with parchment paper. ...

If desired, cut circle shapes with a biscuit cutter or cookie cutter. ...

Bake for about 25-30 minutes (time will vary depending on your chip sizes) or until pumpkin chips begin to curl, edges feel crisp to the touch and are starting to brown.
As simple as that

Boil your spinach,pour out together with its water ,add blanched carrots,baby marrows

Add carb smart beef , and add the carb smart braai spice,seasoned with crushed chilies and salt to taste,add cream and stir

Servings: served with pumpkin chips, you can also fry the ingredients together either with coconut oil or olive oil.

HONEY DIPPED PUMPKIN CHIPS WITH EGG AND VEGETABLE SAUCE:

Ingredients:

Pumpkin chips

4 Eggs

Parsley leaves

Spinach leave

1 full Onion ,

½ glove of Garlic,

 Smoked paprika powder,

Cumin powder,

 Cayenne pepper powder,

 Salt,

Dried herbs.

change your pumpkin game a bit
with cooked eggs and vegetable
sauce! Perfect for a dip dip! And
highly nutritious
Offering, protein, vitamins and
minerals!

Cooking instruction:

To get your pumpkin chips,follow this method:

Preheat the oven to 220°F. Line 2 baking sheets with parchment paper. ...
If desired, cut circle shapes with a biscuit cutter or cookie cutter. …
Roll the cut pumpkins with salt and pepper (if you like Pepper) for taste and dipped in honey preferably for a unique taste!

Bake for about 20-25 minutes

Don't leave it to get too crispy,just have it a bit softly to eat.

Boil your eggs and cut into small sizes and one full for half sizes.

Steam your spinach and add Olive oil, Onion (diced), Garlic, Smoked paprika powder, Cumin powder, Cayenne pepper powder, Salt, Dried herbs, Eggs, and Parsley

For the eggs,break into the cooking pot and let it all steam together ,don't add much water and let it steam for some minutes.

Pour it all out and top with the cut eggs

AFRIQUE VEGGIE SALAD:

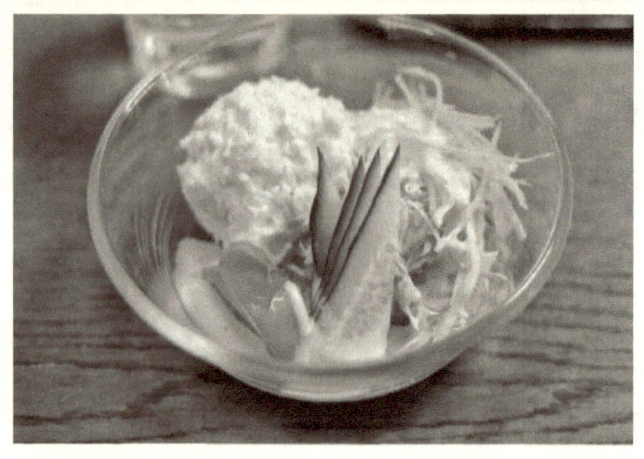

Ingredients:

1 full sizeable cabbage

6-7 carrots

5 pieces of green beans

1 green pepper

Canned sweet corn

Cooked purple bean

Mayonnaise cream

Method:

Wash the cabbage and remove the

outer surface, Chop your

cabbage to desired sizes

Cut the carrots to your desired

sizes

Soak the green beans with hot

water and allow to be edible,and

cut into small pieces

Cut the remaining ingredients and

mix together in a bowl

Pour in your sweat corn as you
mix,let it mix together evenly

Carve out the proportion you can
finish at the time and mix with any
mayonnaise cream.
Preserve the remaining salad in the
refrigerator without. Adding cream.
Serving: serve with rice (preferably)

PINEAPPLE FRIED RICE:

Ingredients:

Rice

Tomato

Cucumber

Chicken Liver

Pineapple

Carrots

Onion

Simple Cooking instruction:

 Cook your plain rice

. Put small oil, fry the liver until

done

After the liver cook, put the rice

. Put Maggie, salt, pepper.

Put maggie, pepper, salt, ketchup

(tomato sauce), soy sauce

(optional)

VEGGIE HONEY BREAD:

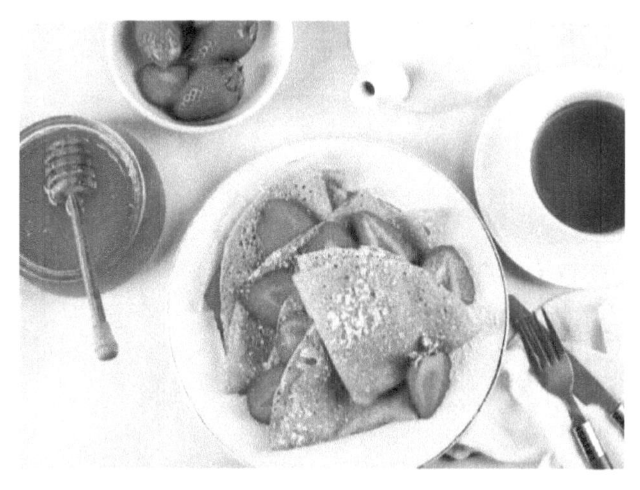

500 grams high protein flour

100 gram sugar

25 grams milk powder

4 items egg yolk

11 grams instant yeast

3 grams bread improver

130 ml liquid milk

100 ml ice water

100 gram butter

1 tsp salt

Almond

Spinach

Fish (mackerel)

Carrots

Honey

Topical ingredients

1 item egg

1/2 tsp salt

1 tbsp milk powder

How to make :

. mix all the dry ingredients add

salt, stir well

. Add milk, water, and egg, stir and knead until smooth

Add almonds, spinach leaves and carrots.
Add fish before adding butter,
Then add honey together with the butter
 Add the butter and knead salt again until smooth and elastic. rest the dough for 15 minutes. the dough is ready to be formed

. cut and weigh the dough 50 gr, round perfectly. rest for another 15 minutes, then form and fill with it.

let it sit for 30 minutes or until it expands. rub the surface with a smear.

5. bake at 180 ° C for 20 minutes or until cooked. remove the heat directly spread with butter and avocado toppings.

SESAME TOPPED AND AVOCADO TOFU SALAD:

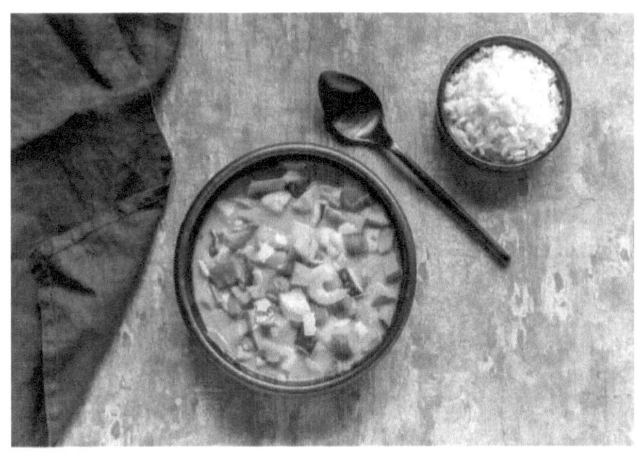

Ingredients:

1 Tablespoon soy sauce

1 Tablespoon almond butter

1/8 tablespoon minced garlic

4 oz tofu, extra firm, thinly sliced

1 cup snow peas, slivered

1/2 tsp sesame seeds

2 Scandinavian crispbread

crackers

½ cut avocado

Directions:

Whisk soy sauce, together with almond butter, avocado and garlic. Toss with tofu and snow peas.

Top with sesame seeds,and serve with crackers.

LOW CAL LAUKI TIKKI:

Ingredients:

1cup of grated Lauki

½ teaspoon of Cumin powder

½ Coriander powder-

½ teaspoon Garam masala

Ajwain- a pinch

Red chilli powder- half

1/3rd cupBread crumbs

Rava/sooji- 1/3rd cup

Salt to taste

Honey to taste

½ lemon

Method:

. Strain the excess water from lauki
and let it dry.

. Add cumin powder, coriander powder, garam masala powder, ajwain, red chilli and salt and mix (mash) well.

 Add lemon juice and honey and mix.

. Mix bread crumbs and rava with lauki and bind it well and make small tikkis out of the mix.

Take a non-stick pan and grease it well with olive oil.

Now place the tikkis on the pan
and toast them on low flame. Flip
them when one side gets brownish
in colour.

 Serve the tikkis hot with green
chutney.

FISH TOMATO SAUCE:

Ingredients:

5 Fresh tomatoes

2 full Onions

1 tomato paste

½ ginger

Vegetable oil

½ garlic

 fish

Curry powder

Salt to taste

Chicken (optional)

Seasonings

Pepper

Chili pepper (optional)

Cooking instruction:

Cook your fresh tomatoes,or just

blend it without cooking (if you

cook it you will still blend it)

Cut your onions to desired shape

Grind the pepper

And grind the ginger

Cut garlic

Meanwhile….your fish is already

cooked with salt and

seasonings,….

Now,place your cooking pot on the

cooking"platform"

Add vegetable oil, enough to fry the

onion and tomatoes….

Put in your onions in the cooking oil

,you should get a "sheeee"

sound…..

Allow just a bit ,to fry small,add the grinded crayfish, and the cut garlic, and Curry powder….

Add pepper to it.

Add the tomato paste and allow it to "fry" till the sour taste disappears,

Meanwhile, keep turning it,so it doesn't burn….add the ginger and turn it all together

Pour in your blended tomatoes and Allow it to cook while turning it, keep tasting it ,and when the "live" taste gets out ,pour in the fish water or chicken water, whichever one you used.

Add salt and other ingredient remaining, check the stew ,if it is moderate don't add water ,if it is thick ,add small water to get it moderate and ok

Continue turning till cooked (Allow the tomatoes to fry well enough before adding any liquid)

Your fish tomato stew is ready! Serve with rice, spaghetti,beans or any cereal crop,can go with anything including fries …..and bread

MUSHROOM-VEGGIE SOUP:

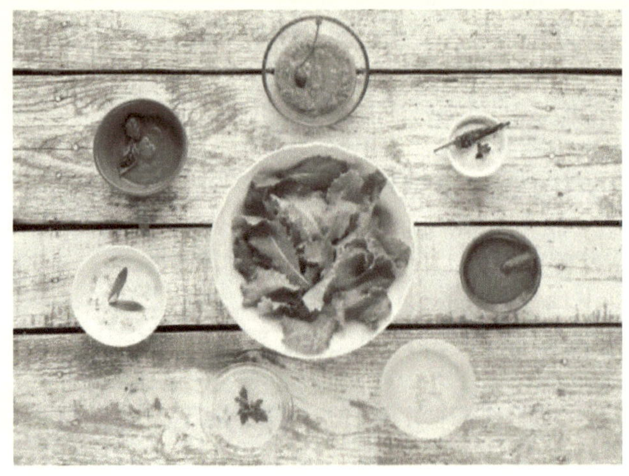

Ingredients:

4 mushroom

Spinach leave

Crayfish

Roasted fish

Salt

Pepper

Broccoli

Onions

Cooking Instruction:

Wash your mushrooms, spinach leaves, broccoli.

Grind your crayfish

Chop your veggie leaves.

Add the grinded crayfish to your cooking pot,add Pepper, and other ingredients (vegetables are last) add salt and seasoning.

Leave it to boil small,

Then add your veggies and turn it all together with onions,

Get the pot down within a minute,so you don't cook off the veggies nutrients.

Tadaaaa your green bowl is ready!

PUMPKIN-AVOCADO GOAT
CHEESE PIZZA:

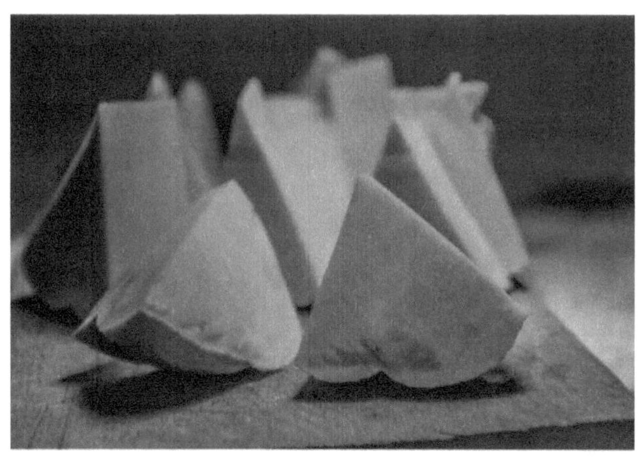

ingredients

4 pieces of crescent-cut pumpkin
5 Fresh cut avocado
Whole grain or reg. pizza crust
3c thinly sliced fuji apples (about 8
oz)
1c(4 oz)crumbled goat cheese
2tsp fresh thyme
1T olive oil
2tsp dijon mustard
1tsp fresh lemon juice

1-2 tablespoon of honey
2c baby arugula
3T chopped pecans, toasted

Instruction;

Preheat the oven to 450°.
Place pizza crust on a baking sheet
coated with cooking spray.

Arrange pumpkin slices evenly
over pizza crust; top with cheese.
Sprinkle thyme evenly over
cheese.
Bake at 450° for 8 minutes or until
the cheese melts and begins to
brown.

Combine oil and remaining
ingredients with honey) in a

medium bowl, stirring with a whisk
including avocados

 Add arugula; toss gently to coat.
Sprinkle pecans evenly over pizza;
top with avocado mixture. Cut
pizza desirably.

VEGGIE BLACK BEAN CHILI AND
CORNBREAD:

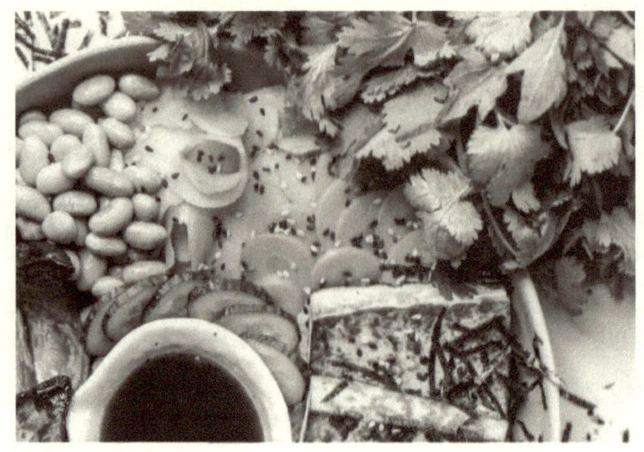

Ingredients:

5 cups Cornbread or Jalapeno
Cornbread cut into 1-inch cubes
5 cups 1-inch toasted sourdough
cubes
2 tablespoons olive oil
2 cups finely chopped yellow onion
2 large garlic cloves, minced
1½ cups cubanelle peppers,
seeded and finely diced
1 cup finely chopped celery

Sea salt and freshly ground black
pepper, to taste
2 lightly beaten eggs
1 cup chicken, turkey or vegetable
stock
tbsp olive oil
2 red onions, finely chopped
1 carrot, chopped
1 stalk celery, chopped
2 tsp ground cumin
1 ½ tsp ground coriander
1 tsp dried crushed oregano
½ heaped tsp ground allspice
(optional if you don't have it but it
does add something special to the
soup)
1 ancho chilli (a dried poblano
chilli) or other mild, fruity-tasting
dried chilli

400 ml vegetable stock (keep more
handy in case you find you want it
soupier)
1 x 400g tin good quality chopped
tomatoes (I like Cirio)
1 tbsp sundried tomato paste or
regular tomato paste
½ aubergine/eggplant, small cubes
2 x 400 g tins black beans, drained
but not rinsed
20 g packet leaf coriander,
chopped just before using
1 lime, halved

This is an easy and vegetable
loaded take on traditional chili.
Serve with white or brown basmati
rice or – my favourite – cornbread.
This recipe easily doubles for
freezing or parties.

Heat the olive oil in a large, lidded saucepan. Saute the onions over a low heat until translucent, about four minutes (you can sauté in a little bit of vegetable stock rather than the oil).

Stir in the other vegetables, garlic, oregano, cumin, coriander, allspice and ancho chilli, and sauté for one minute before adding the stock, tomatoes, tomato paste, aubergine/eggplant and beans.

Bring to the boil, then turn down to simmer. Allow to bubble away for 20 minutes before stirring in chopped coriander (save a little for garnish), juice from half of the lime, and any seasoning.

.

 Fish out the chilli and serve the black bean chilli topped with crème fraiche/sour cream, extra lime and a big wedge of cornbread.

.

Preheat the oven to 350 degrees. Combine the cornbread and bread cubes in a large bowl. Set aside. Heat the oil in a large skillet. Add

the onions and sauté over a

medium heat until softened, about

8 minutes. Add the garlic and sauté

for another 5 minutes.

Add the peppers and celery and

cook stirring, until they are tender

but still crisp. Season with salt and
pepper and set aside to cool
slightly.

Add the onion mixture to the
cornbread and mix well. Add the
eggs and enough stock to lightly
moisten the stuffing.

Lightly press the stuffing into a
greased 10x15-inch baking pan.
Cover with foil. Put the stuffing pan
into a larger high-sided pan to
make a bain-marie. Fill the larger
pan halfway with boiling water and
bake for 50 minutes.

AVOCADO PEANUT BUTTER SMOOTHIE:

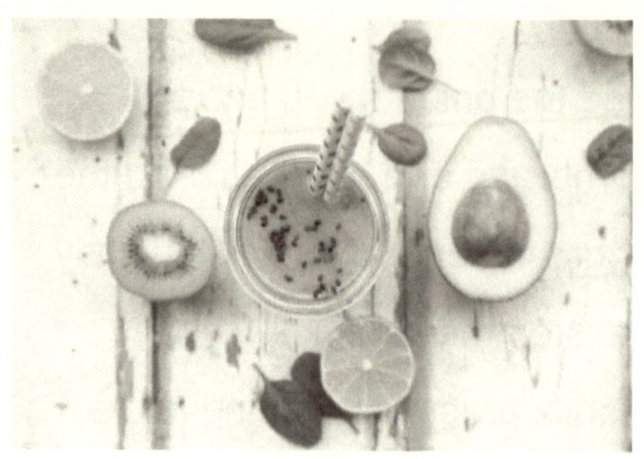

Ingredients:

2 sliced avocado pear
1/2 cup 1% low-fat milk.
1/2 cup vanilla fat-free yogurt.
2 tablespoons ground golden flaxseed.
1 tablespoon creamy peanut butter.
1 teaspoon honey.

1 cup Unsweetened Coconut Milk

2 Tbsp Peanut Butter

2 Tbsp ground Flaxseed Meal

1 tsp Vanilla extract

 1 handful of almond

1 tablespoon of powdered soyabeans

Instruction:

Slice avocado and blend it together with honey

Blend other ingredients until smooth and add almonds, stir evenly and enjoy!

Tadaaaa!

PEANUT AND PUMPKIN MUFFINS:

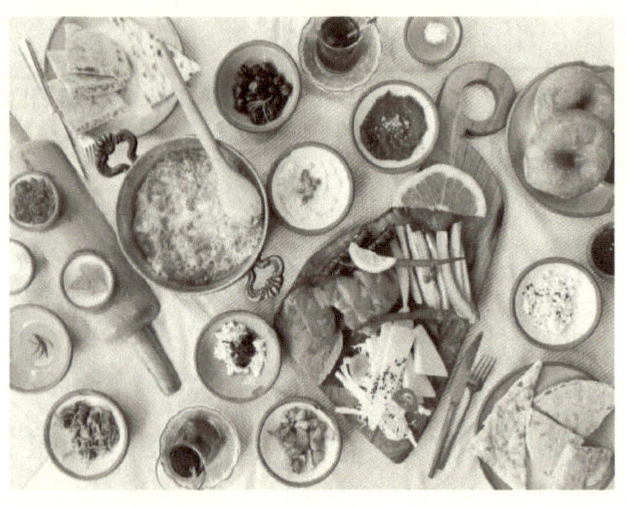

Total Time
37 mins

Calories: 90kcal

Ingredients:

1 tablespoon large flake oats

1 tbsp pumpkin seeds

2 tbsp coarsely chopped peanuts

1 tbsp brown sugar

1 cup all purpose flour

3/4 cup whole wheat flour

1 1/4 cups sugar

½ tbsp baking powder

1 1/2 tsp chinese five spice powder

⅓ tsp salt

1 cup unsweetened canned pumpkin

1/2 c peanut oil

1/3 cup water

2 eggs

1 tsp vanilla

1/3 cup peanut butter

Instructions

Preheat the oven to 375 F. Lightly grease a muffin pan.

Combine oats, pumpkin seeds, peanuts and brown sugar in a small bowl and set aside.

In a large bowl, stir flour with sugar, baking powder, five-spice powder and salt. In a medium bowl, whisk pumpkin with oil, water, eggs and vanilla.
 Whisk in peanut butter.
Pour onto flour mixture and stir until combined.

Spoon batter into prepared muffins pan and sprinkle with topping.
 Bake for 22 minutes or until the tester comes out clean. Let cool in the pan for 5 minutes then transfer to a rack to cool.
Ready to serve ,

BAKED PUMPKIN-PEAS HONEY COOKIES:

Ingredients:

1 cup flour

2 teaspoon vanilla flavour

1 teaspoon sugar

2 eggs

2 tablespoon of milk

3-4 tablespoon of honey

added baking powder

Peas

2tablespoon of butter (measure enough for the dough)

Pumpkin (small square cookie sizes or any of your preferred shape and sizes)

Instruction:

Cut out your pumpkins into your desired shape and sizes.

Prepare your dough by:

Pour in your flour into a bowl ,add sugar, vanilla flavour and baking powder,stir well and add milk(liquid or powder)

Add butter and enough honey

Stir gently and easily till smooth...

Whisk your eggs and pour into the bowl,

Prepare your dough very well

Next step:

You can either choose to roll your dough or either use this step, which is recommended for this;

As your dough is ready in its form in your bowl,all you have to do now is to coat evenly to your sliced pumpkin,

For the pumpkin to bake well,you can bake it differently or ,as it is still fresh coat with your honey dough and let it have enough mass.

Stuff or pierce with your peas

Then bake until done enough!

HEALTHY HOME HONEY BEVERAGE:

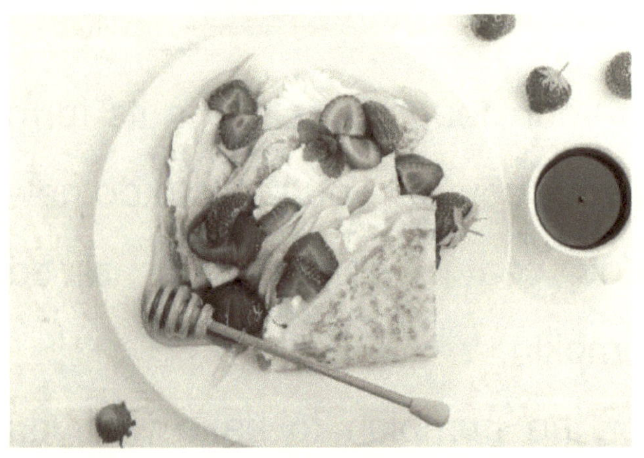

Honey

3 cups Cocoa powder

2cups of Cocoa Starch

2teaspoon Egg yolk

2teaspoon Baking

Sugar 1 and half cup

Milk flavor 2sachets

Vanilla flavor 2teaspoon

Instruction:

pour corn starch inside the cocoa
powder and stir until the cornstarch
and cocoa powder are properly
mixed .

Add your sugar.

Add milk flavor and stir.

Add powder egg yolk.

Add Baking Soda.

Add Vanilla flavor and keep stirring, stir all corners to enable the ingredient mix nicely.
Store and preserve.
Add honey anytime you want to drink it.

BORLOTTI BEAN MOLE WITH ROASTED YAM AND SPINACH:

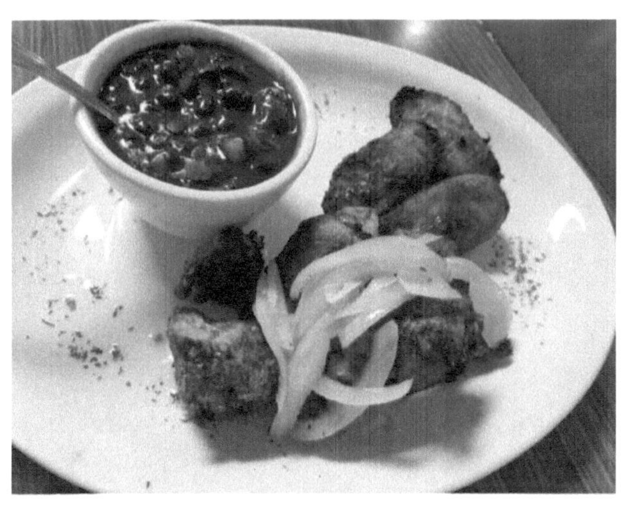

Ingredients:

4 cups cooked borlotti / cranberry
beans

About 7 ounces peeled yam ,   cut
into 2 cm or 3/4-inch cubes)
olive oil for roasting the yam

4 – 5 big leaves of kale (3 1/2
ounces) [I used much more than
this.]
2 tablespoons butter [If you switch
this to olive oil or coconut oil then
the recipe is vegan.]

1 medium onion, chopped
2 – 4 red jalapeno chiles, halved,
seeded, and chopped.

2 garlic cloves, chopped
1 pound of fresh plum tomatoes,
chopped or 14-ounce can
2 teaspoons paprika

1 ounce of almonds, dark roasted and finely ground [use pre-ground almonds and then toast the meal in a small skillet.]

2 ounces dark 70% dark chocolate, broken into pieces [I used 85% chocolate, and the dish was definitely sweet enough]

1 tsp. salt

 Garden eggs

 Instructions:

Preheat the oven to 180C / 350F.

Roast the Yam: Cut the yam flesh into good-sized chunks, about 2 cm or 3/4-inch squares, place them in a roasting pan and toss with olive oil and rub little salt all over the yam.

Roast them in the oven for about 20 minutes or till done to your desired result or until caramelized on the outside but still firm.

Reduce the oven temperature to 130C/ 250F / Gas mark 1/2. Without removing the central stem, cut the kale across the leaf into 2cm / 3/4-inch slices.

Melt the butter into an oven-proof casserole dish (pot) and fry the onion and chilies gently over a low to medium heat for 20-30 minutes, until caramelized.

Add the garlic and fry for three minutes more. Add the tomatoes and paprika, bring to a boil, reduce the heat and simmer gently for 15 minutes,simmer the spinach as well and bring out separately.

Add the ground almonds, chocolate, , borlotti beans, kale,

and salt. Stir until the chocolate has melted.

Cover the casserole and put it in the oven to cook gently until done.

Then serve with the roasted yam mixed together with the beans bowl and topped with the cooked spinach and top with your cut garden eggs.

Serves 4

YAM PEPPERED VEGGIE SOUP:

Ingredients

Yam

Beef (cow hump & Brisket bone)

 the best to use are assorted meat:

Shaki (cow tripe)

Kidney

Heart

Liver

Fuku

animal skin (cow or,goat or pork)

6pieces seeds Calabash nutmeg,

Scent leaves

Onions

Scotch bonnet and Chilli Pepper

Peppersoup spice

2 big seasoning cubes

Salt (to taste)

Before you cook the Yam Pepper

Soup

Peel and cut the yam tuber into

medium cubes. Rinse and set

aside.

Peel, roast and grind the Calabash

seeds with a dry mill or pound in

mortar.(grind,)

Slice the onions, scent leaves and grind the pepper.

Cut the beef into bite sizes.

Method

Put the meat in a pot, add the seasoning cubes and part of the onions (diced).

Pour water to cover the contents and start cooking. Keep an eye on it and top up the water when necessary.

After 30 mins - 45 mins, depending on the type of meat. Shaki will take a longer time to cook.

Add yam cubes, the second part of onions (diced), salt and continue cooking.

Add water to the same level as the contents of the pot if necessary.

When the yam is soft and a little porridge starts to form, add the grinded pepper, chilli pepper, pepper soup spice and the scent leaves.

Stir, cover and cook for 5mins and it is done!

Serve hot with your favourite smoothie!

OKRO SOUP:

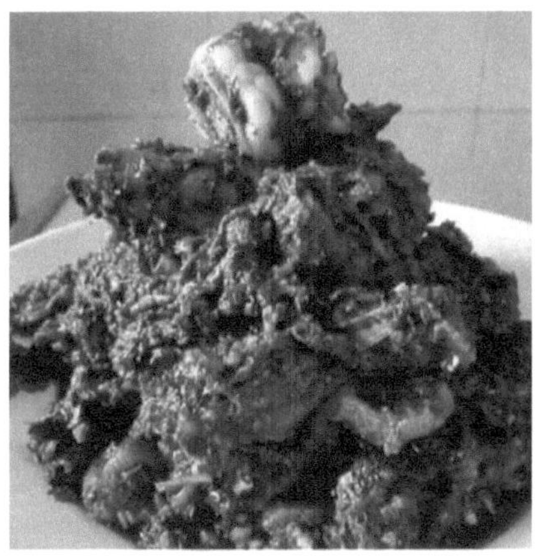

Ingredients:

-Okro (chopped)

-Pumpkin leaves (chopped)

-Fresh pepper (blended

-Chicken (any meat can serve)

-Crayfish

-Palm oil(red oil/)

-Seasoning Cubes

-Salt

-Roasted fish

-pounded- locust bean

Cooking Instruction:

Cook the chicken and the smoked fish. But if you are using beef, make sure that the meat is almost done before you add the smoked fish.

Add seasoning cubes and salt to taste.

When the meat is done, pour in your pounded pepper, locust bean and crayfish, add palm oil, check if there is need to add another seasoning cubes and salt, cover and let it cook for about 2-3 minutes.

Add the chopped okro and vegetable. Cover for about 1 min or less and turn off the light.

Make sure you remove the pot from the heated cooker to a cooler surface so that the vegetables will not be over cooked

Serve with semovita or any of your preferred

MILLET-GINGER POTATO MILK SMOOTHIE:

Ingredients:

Millet

Potatoes

Ginger

Cloves

Dry pepper little

Sugar to taste

Instruction:

Grind ur Millet aside

Grind main ingredient aside

Pour boiling water in to your Millet

mix like pap (semi-liquid)add your

Ginger mix and leave it for about

8 hours

 you will see water on top of it

remove the water gently and use it

to sieve it ,

add sugar and put in fridge

It should be left overnight (grinded millet)before filter

Pour in milk whenever you want to drink it and serve cold!

Goes with anything good!

FRIED VEGGIE MACKEREL:

Ingredients:

Mackerel fish

Carrots

Sesame dressing

Cabbage

Soy sauce.

Pepper

Salt

Instructions;

Cut the mackerel into bite-sized pieces

Cut the carrot and cabbage into small pieces.

Preparing the seasoning blend;

Mix together the sesame dressing and soy sauce in a bowl.

Seasoning the ingredients;
Add the defrosted mackerel, carrot, and cabbage to the bowl containing the seasoning blend and mix thoroughly so that the seasonings coat the ingredients.

Stir-frying

Add oil to frying pan over medium heat.
Once the frying pan is hot, add the seasoned mackerel and vegetables

along with the seasoning blend and cook for 3-4 minutes or until the sides of the mackerel are golden brown.

AVOCADO TOPPED BREADFRUIT:

Serving: 3

Ingredients:

5 cups of breadfruit

1 teaspoon pepper

1-½ teaspoon salt

2 tablespoon olive oil (any oil/if you don't have read oil,which is palm oil,you can improvise,)

2 fresh tomatoes

1 onion

Crayfish/roasted fish

Seasoning

1 tablespoon of honey

Meat

Cooking Instruction:

Naturally,this breadfruit is yummy,it has such an amazing taste that's superb.

Wash your breadfruit and pour in to your cooking pot

So,start off by cooking the breadfruit,it usually takes time to cook, when it is done it should be in porridge form.

Now get your ingredients ready, Tomatoes should be sliced, onion too,get your roasted fish ready,or fresh fish whichever one you prefer

If you're using fresh fish,cook with seasoning and keep,you only pour in the fish water or meat water to the pot .

when the breadfruit gets like beans,taste and check you should know when it is ready,add all the ingredients,oil first and honey last.

If you're cooking with meat,pour in the meat's water ,and don't let the food get solid ,you should get it down when it is still a bit watery because when it gets cold ,it congeles.

As easy as that ! It isn't hard to make and very delicious! With high nutrients

Top your breadfruit plate with avocados sliced

RED-OILED PUMPKIN:

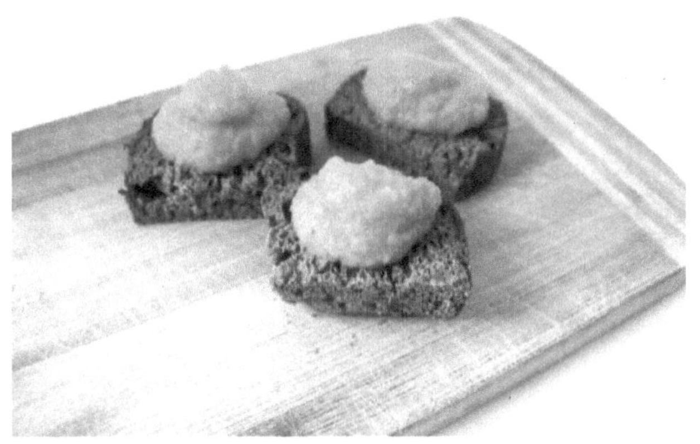

Ingredients:

Pumpkin

Cauliflower

red oil (palm oil)or olive/vegetable

oil

Salt

Onions

Garlic cloves

Crayfish

Tomato (optional)

Scent leaves

Garden eggs

Cooking Instruction:

Cut pumpkin to your desired sizes and shapes and a portion you can consume

Boil with water separately….
When done ,keep it aside and begin your fry……

Slice onions and garlic,
Cut scent leaves,
Grind or blend your crayfish
Have your garden eggs chopped,get ready pepper, seasoning, and Salt…

Place your frying pan on the fire,and add palm oil/red oil, leave a bit and pour in enough onions , and a little garlic, turn it and add pepper and other ingredients,stir with the red oil…... for the red oil fry,it usually chokes when heating so put on a face mask or nose mask whichever one !

The aroma of the fry is appetising though,so watch it so it doesn't get burned, put enough onions ok

Add scent leaves,and get it down!
Add cauliflower to your taste!

Tadaaaa your plain cooked pumpkin is ready to be served with oil onion sauce

Now,if you are not using red oil,use any other oil, and that's where tomato comes in, tomato should be sliced into small sizes..

The red oil sauce can be taken with yam! And it is very yummy and delicious!

It can also serve white rice,red oil is versatile.

Take your cooked pumpkin,you can either choose to scrape it all to your plate and then pour in the sauce and enjoy with cauliflower

Or take a spoonful of the sauce and topped to the pumpkin for every " intake"

RIPPED ROASTED PLANTAIN AND PORRIDGE BEANS:

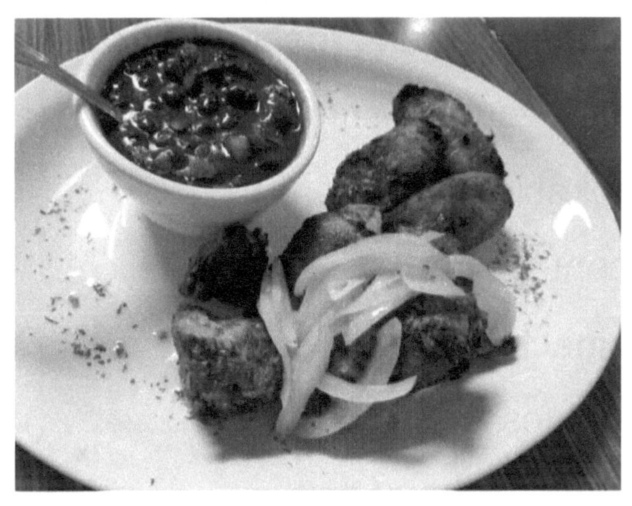

change your bean game with this salivating served -hot bean and plantain porridge

Servings :
Serves 2 -3

Ingredients:

4 cups of Beans (depending on the bean you're using,but let it be a cookable tasteful one)

Scent leaves

Spinach leaves

3 onions

2-3 teaspoon of salt

3-4 teaspoon of Pepper

Seasoning cubes

4 ripe plantain

Red oil/palm oil (enough to fry)

2-3 medium sized garden egg

Cooking Instruction:

Cook beans with salt and garlic
only, when done set aside and
commence the main course+sauce

Roast ripen plantains and do not
cut it yet, roast till the outer body
gets crispy and hardened

Put your red oil in your frying
pan,the oil should be much,so it
can serve better..,...

Slice onions and garlic, don't let the
oil fry deep,add garlic and scent
leaves,add   salt   and   pepper

enough,if you like Pepper add onions and bring the pan down.

While the beans is still hot,add chopped spinach,or if you love it raw ,just chop it and hover all over your complete plate

So this is how it is done,
Now, using your hand or knife ,divide the plantain little by little pour in the beans in the bowl,and add your red oil onion sauce then top your spinach
Top garden eggs chopped or sliced

Mix it all together and enjoy! Add extra live Fresh onions

APPLE PEANUT BUTTER BITE:

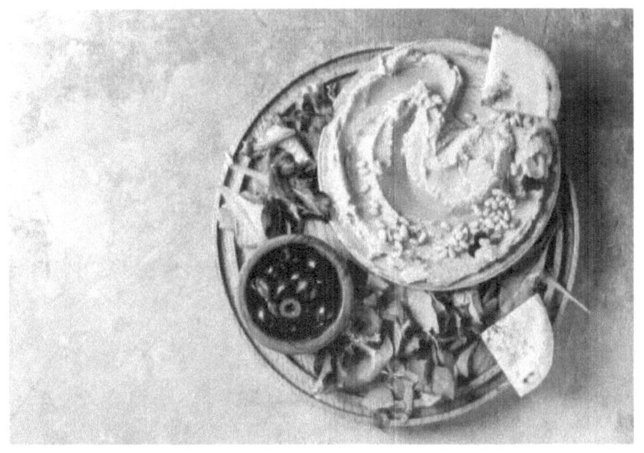

Ingredients:

2 medium Apples

¼ Cup creamy nut butter (anyone)

¾ cup baking chocolate

½ tablespoon coconut oil

¼ milk (liquid/semi/solid)

Instruction:

Cover baking sheet with parchment paper,

Slice each Apple into thin slices or crescent, arrange on the baking sheet.

Now,spread peanut butter in each slice and cover each slice with another slice just like a sandwich or hamburger.

Place in the freezer for Upto 30 Minutes until frozen

place coconut oil in a microwave safe bowl and wave until melted.

Stir in the chocolate, and milk ,it could be solid or semi liquid continue to microwave until smooth

.

Use a fork to cover each Apple bite in chocolate milk ,then place back on the sheet .

Freeze for one hour and enjoy your crunchy bite!

Thaw for a few mins before eating

Yield: 10

Serving:2 b

Good source of protein and fibre!

HONEY-DIPPED CABBAGE CHEESE PLUMS:

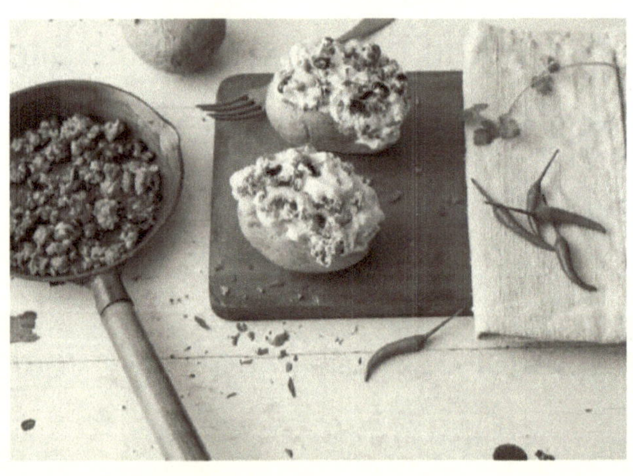

Ingredients:

3 Plums, halved & pitted

1 dash Olive oil, for drizzling

1 tablespoon Sugar

 1 tablespoon of butter

1 dash chopped cabbage

1 dash Salt & pepper

1 dash Fresh-chopped basil, for topping

7 ounces Goat cheese

1 dash Chopped pistachios & balsamic vinegar, for garnish

1 tablespoon honey

 1 handful of peanuts

Preparation;

Preheat the oven to 400 degrees. Place plums side by side,cut-side up on a foil-lined sheet pan.

Drizzle with coconut oil and
sprinkle with sugar, salt and pepper
and coat with honey and butter
Mix the honey and butter in a
separate bowl with a little milk and
chopped cabbage

Dip in your peanuts to the it as
many as you can,or just take a
handful of chopped peanuts and
rub all over it

Top with fresh-chopped basil, and
bake for 15 minutes.

When cooled, spread 1 ounce of
goat cheese on each half, topping
with chopped pistachios &
balsamic vinegar.
Enjoy your brown Cheese!

VEGGIE GRILLED SWEET POTATO AND COCONUT RICE:

Ingredients:

3 sweet potatoes cut into 1/2 inch
wedges
2 tbsp extra virgin olive oil
1/2 tsp Tajin or to taste
1 Big Coconut.(if you can't get the
coconut Fruit itself use about
1 coconut milk can
3 cups of rice
Fresh ground tomatoes (500ml)

2 Tablespoons (tomato paste) (tin tomato)
Chicken (2KG)
1 cup of sliced onions
3 seasoning cubes
Half teaspoon of chicken spice
Vegetable oil half cup (150ml)
Teaspoon ground ginger.
Half teaspoon of ground garlic

Cooking Instructions:

Place the potatoes in a large saucepan and cover with water. Bring to a boil, cover and simmer for 4 minutes until crisp tender. Drain well and dry very well. Toss with olive oil and tajin.

Grill over medium heat, covered,
for 10 or so minutes or until tender
with grill marks.

'

 making coconut rice;

 start by breaking and de-shelling

the cocoanut and grind (sort of

grind) the coconut with a grater, the

idea is to squeeze out the milk from

the main coconut,you can just use

an already made coconut milk but

this one is way better

Normally you grate the coconut
with a grater and then add a cup of
water or two and then squeeze out
the coconut milk . Filter the

squeezed out milk and set aside in
a bowl

-Parboil three cups of rice, grind
the tomatoes/peppers (you need
about 500ml), your blender should
be calibrated, or you can slice the
tomatoes if you like.

Also parboil the chicken with all the
necessary ingredients (half cup of
sliced onions, 2 seasonings cubes,
Salt, and half teaspoon of chicken
spice), add a cup of water.

Allow cooking till it is soft, around
10-15 minutes.

Pick the chicken with a kitchen fork
and deep fry, set aside the stock.

-Set your cooking pot on heat, add a half-cup (150ml) of vegetable oil, allow heating for at least 90 seconds before adding the tomatoes.
Now fry and stir the tomatoes for the next 10-15 minutes till it is dried.

Add the chicken stock once you are done with frying the tomatoes, also add the coconut milk.

Add a seasoning cube, add more salt to taste. Allow boiling before adding the rice, then the remaining half cup of sliced onions.

Cook for the next twenty to forty minutes until the rice is soft and ready to serve.

Serve with your grilled potatoes and chicken (optional)

RASPBERRY FILLED MERINGUES AND BLUEBERRY SAUCE:

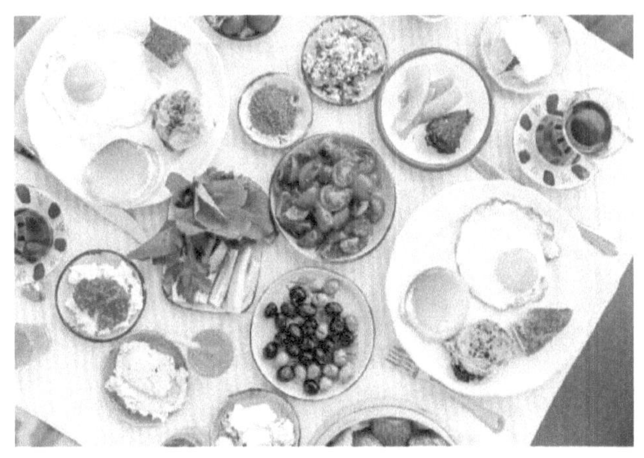

Ingredients

For the meringues;
3   Egg white(s)
150gWhite caster sugar
1 teaspoon   Rose water
1 teaspoon   Pink food colouring

150gRaspberries
2 tablespoon   Icing sugar
150ml   Double cream

blueberry sauce;

ingredients

2 cups frozen (or fresh) blueberries
1/3 cup water
1/4 cup granulated sugar (white or
coconut is fine -- a natural
granulated sweetener may be used
that measures 1:1 with sugar)
2 tablespoons lemon juice (or
orange juice)
1 1/2 tablespoons cornstarch (corn
flour) mixed with 2 tablespoons
water

instructions

Combine the blueberries, water,
sugar, lemon juice and water in a

small-sized saucepan over medium-high heat.

Bring to a boil; lower heat and gently simmer.
Combine the cornstarch with the extra water until dissolved and stir it into the blueberries. Continue to simmer while stirring occasionally, until the sauce begins to thicken and coats the back of a metal spoon..

Preheat the oven to 120°c (fan 100°c, gas mark ½).

Beat the egg whites in a clean, dry bowl until the whites double in volume and hold peaks.

While the whisk is still running add the sugar a tablespoon at a time, until all the sugar is added and the whites are glossy and hold a stiff peak.

Fold in the rose water. Be careful not to over beat.

On two baking trays place a dot of the meringue mixture in each corner of the baking trays, then stick a piece of baking paper onto the baking tray. This will stop the paper from moving around when you pipe on the meringues.

Pour about 1 tsp of the pink food colouring onto a saucer and use a wide pastry brush to brush a line of the colouring up the inside of a

piping bag. Spoon the meringue
mix into the bag.

Pipe the meringue into 3.5cm wide
swirls or drop the mixture using a
teaspoon.

Bake for 90 minutes until they are
crisp and lift off the paper easily.
Turn off the oven and leave to cool
in the oven with the door ajar for
another hour or even overnight.

To make the raspberry coulis for
the filling: Put the raspberries and 1
tbsp icing sugar into the bowl of a
food processor and blend to a
purée.

Set a sieve over a clean bowl and rub the purée through to remove the raspberry pips.

To serve, whisk the cream and remaining icing sugar until softly peaked. Swirl in the raspberry coulis. Spoon or pipe the cream onto half the meringues and sandwich with the remaining meringues.

Serve with the blueberry sauce!

HONEYED PAWPAW FETA:

Ingredients:

Three ripen cut papaya
2 tablespoon honey
Salt and freshly cracked pepper to taste
4 ounces feta cheese
2 red tomatoes,
1 cup basil leaves
2 tablespoons olive oil
2 teaspoons balsamic vinegar

Instruction:

, cut the pawpaw in half squares. Remove the seeds Cut into thin slices square wise.

Softly Sprinkle tomatoes and pawpaw with salt and pepper and drizzle with olive oil and balsamic vinegar and fresh honey

Cut the feta into thin slices. Lay the pawpaw, feta, and basil in stacks on plates,top all body with honey

AVOCADO-COCONUT MILK:

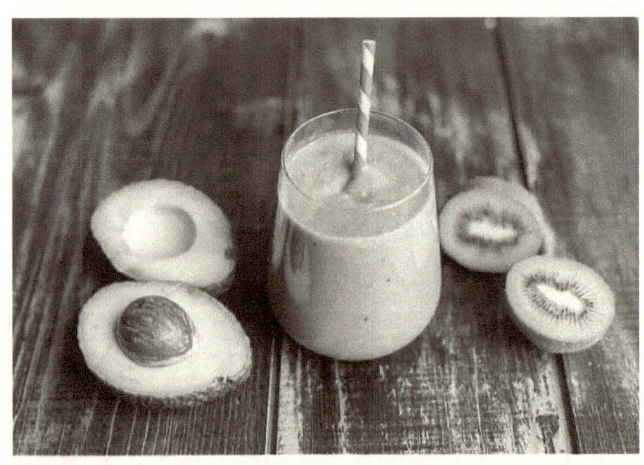

try out this yummy avocado and coconut milk smoothie recipe;

Ingredients:

1 cup coconut milk
2-3 full avocado
½ cup liquid milk
1teaspoon of sugar to taste
⅓ cup soya bean (powdered/or about 3 tablespoon) this is optional
Apple Cider vinegar (taste to know when enough)

Instruction:

Peel out avocados, and remove the entire fruit,blend together with liquid milk,sugar, soyabean and apple cider until smooth enough

Pour in the coconut milk and blend together for an even smoothie,add water only if necessary or as you desire.

You're gonna love the taste! So great!
Serve chilled, anything can go with it.

CHOCOLATE HONEY SOYA MILK:

blend in your chocolate, honey and milk with (to) soya bean

Ingredients:

Chocolate
3-4 tablespoon honey
Liquid milk (enough)
Sugar to taste
Powdered soya bean

Instruction:
Blend your ingredients together
with a little water,
Serve chilled,goes with pretty much
anything.

CARROT AND CABBAGE MILK MIX:

Ingredients:

7-8 medium sized sweet carrots

½   -one   ounce   of   cabbage
-chopped

½   ginger   clove(blended-water
strained out)

 1 tin liquid milk

 1 teaspoon sugar

  Vanilla flavour

Instruction:

Scrape the carrots to smoothened
and fresh
Place in a blender, and blend .
Bring out in a cup or bowl with its
water together.
Place the chopped cabbage in the
blender and puree until smooth
Grind or blend ginger and filter the
liquid,that's the only thing you need
from it.

In a bowl or cup ,pour out the blended mixtures add the milk and sugar and stir until even
Add vanilla flavour and stir

It shouldn't be watery,but should be semi-liquid enough to be held by your spoon

Put in the cup or bowl into the freezer, freezer till frozen

Enjoy! It can be a topping or filler for your bread and rolls

ROASTED CUCUMBER AND YOGHURT PASTA:

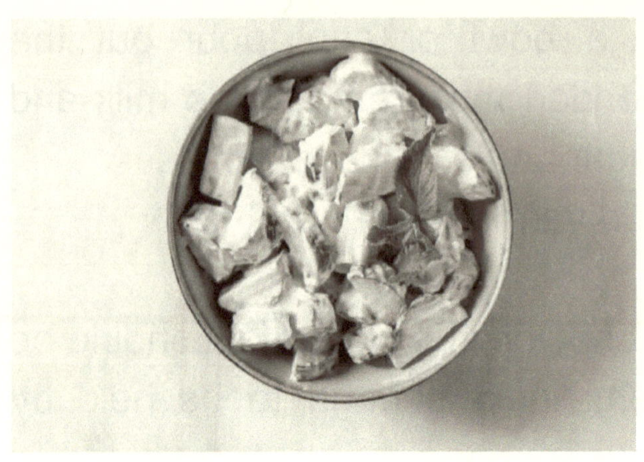

Ingredients:

10,5 oz / 300 g cucumber
Seasoning
3 tablespoon olive oil
1,5 tablespoon lemon juice
1 ½ teaspoon liquid sweetener
1 ½ teaspoon ground cumin
1 teaspoon ground coriander
1/2 tsp salt
1/4 tsp cayenne pepper
Coconut yogurt sauce

1/2 cup unsweetened natural flavored coconut yogurt
1 tsp lemon juice
1/4 tsp salt
black pepper
Other ingredients
Pasta for 4
~1/2 cup fresh mint
~1/4 cup grated vegan parmesan
black pepper to taste
dried chili flakes to taste

Instruction:

Preheat oven
Rinse and dry cucumbers and chop large into medium sized

Mix the seasoning ingredients and use about 1/2 of the sauce to coat the cucumbers.

Leave the rest of the seasoning to serve with pasta.

Roast cucumbers on a baking sheet for about 5 min

Mix coconut yogurt ingredients.
Cook pasta according to instructions.
Serve pasta with roasted cucumbers, yogurt sauce, rest of the seasoning mix, fresh mint, vegan parmesan, black pepper and chili flakes.

PASTA AND BEANS WITH COCONUT YOGHURT DRESSING:

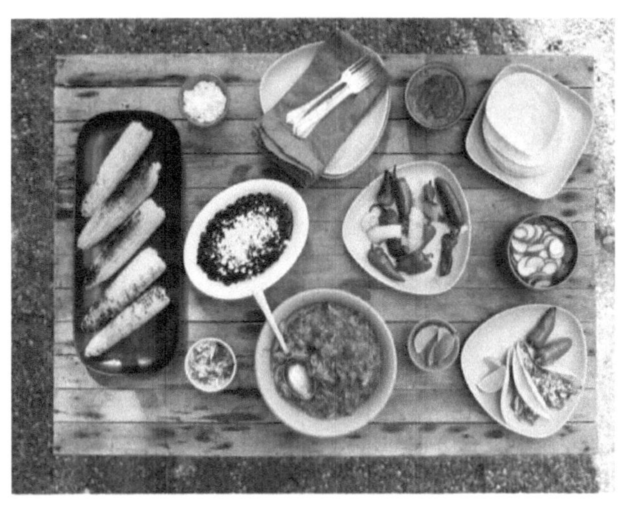

Ingredients:

3 cups of beans

Seasoning

3 tablespoon olive oil

1,5 tablespoon lemon juice

1 ½ teaspoon liquid sweetener

1 ½ teaspoon ground cumin

1 teaspoon ground coriander
1/2 tsp salt
1/4 tsp cayenne pepper
Coconut yogurt sauce
1/2 cup unsweetened natural flavored coconut yogurt
1 tsp lemon juice
1/4 tsp salt
black pepper
Other ingredients
Pasta for 4
~1/2 cup fresh mint
~1/4 cup grated vegan parmesan
black pepper to taste
dried chili flakes to taste

Cooking Instruction;

Cooking the Beans:

put beans in a pot, cover them with water, bring them up to a boil, and then cover the pot and turn off the heat. Let them sit for at least a half an hour in the hot water, drain them, and rinse.

Now is time for the main cooking

Turn on the heat and pour in sizeable amount of water

After about 30 minutes to an hour, once your beans are tender and soft enough, turn off the heat, and season the cooking liquid to taste.

This is where you salt heavily and add any acidic ingredients, like tomatoes or lemon juice. When you're tasting for seasoning, you want to taste the broth rather than the beans themselves,

which is why it's important to let them hang out in their cooking liquid for a half an hour before eating them.

If you're planning on packing them up and storing them for later use, let them cool completely in their cooking liquid beforehand.

Now slice your onions, shallots, garlic, and chiles. Or maybe some fresh herbs like rosemary, sage, bay leaves, and thyme.

And it all to your beans
This is where the flavor really starts to build. Salt the liquid again

(lightly) after about an hour of simmering.

Now the beans is done ,set aside and commence cooking the pasta

Cook pasta as instructed,and cook the seasoning ingredients to a sauce

Mix the yoghurt dressing,you can have it chilled!

Serve pasta alongside with your beans and yoghurt sauce dressing

Enjoy!

Serves many

TOMATO-SAUCE RICE AND BEANS:

Ingredients:

1 ½ cups of beans

2½cups of rice (parboiled/drained)

3-4 fresh tomatoes

 Tomato pasta (optional)

1 clove garlic

ginger

2 Onions

Seasonings

1 teaspoon Curry powder

1-2 teaspoon of salt to taste

Grinded black pepper

Fish or meat

Olive oil/vegetable oil

Cooking Instruction:
There's no hard part here, Because it is all simple,

All you have to do is cook your Beans (many beans are naturally sweetened, like the brown Beans,honey beans etc) so cook beans with its procedures with only salt ,add garlic and ginger to it if desired.

Cook white rice with salt to taste and just sprinkle a little seasoning to the white rice,no added ingredients.

Now the main part is the tomato sauce/stew....

slice your onions, garlic and blend
Tomatoes,
Grind the ginger and Pepper
If you're using fish to serve,pour in
the fish/meat water

Now place your pot/pan on the
heat pour in your cooking oil,leave
to heat for sometime

Add your sliced onions and stir,add
curry powder,for a great taste and
aroma!

Put garlic and ginger,allow to fry a
little while stirring it.

Pour in blended tomatoes (if you're
also using tomato paste,put in

tomato paste first before the blended fresh tomatoes)

Stir gently and allow the tomato to fry ,add salt and other seasoning and Pepper,stir all through, taste the stew ,if the tomato loosen it's natural taste then it is done .

Add a little water and stir , the stew should be kind of thick,or anyhow you like it!

Take a proportion of beans topped to the rice,or placed aside
Using your spoon,add the needed quantity of tomato stew

Serve hot! With your favourite smoothie or fruit juice

BANANA-AVOCADO VEGGIE BOWL:

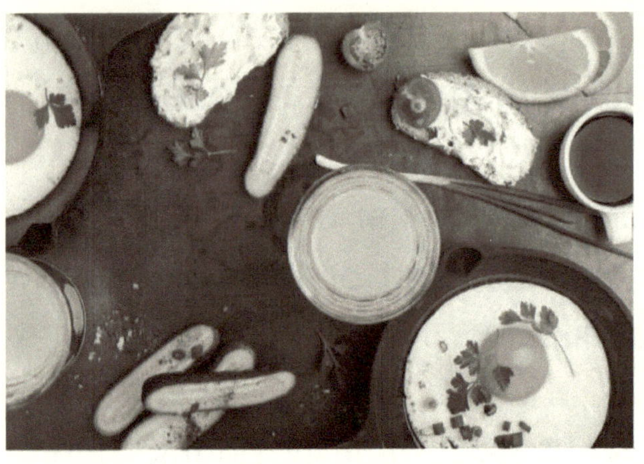

1 medium sized avocado pear
2 frozen bananas, peeled
2 kiwis, peeled
1 cup clean pineapple chunks
1 cup unsweetened almond
milk

1 tablespoon honey
 1 teaspoon lemon juice
2 teaspoons blue spirulina
powder
½ cup clean blueberries
½ small Fuji apple, thinly
sliced and cut into 1-inch
flower shapes
Fresh spinach leave(if desired)

Instructions:

Mix your bananas, avocado,and
kiwis, pineapple, almond milk,
honey, and added lemon juice and
spirulina in a blender,blend
excessively till it is smooth, about
3 minutes.

Freeze….

Divide the smoothie among 2 bowls. pinnacle with blueberries and apples,

Serve chilled! Or well as you desire.

BLACK BEAN BURRITOS AND CUCUMBER FILLINGS:

Ingredients:
1 dash Fresh-chopped basil
300 g cucumber
1 Tbsp olive oil
1 medium onion, chopped
2 tsp minced garlic

16 oz baby bella mushrooms, sliced

4 oz pumpkin roughly chopped

1 can black beans, rinsed and drained

1 tsp chili powder

1/2 teaspoon cumin

 salt, to taste

1.5 cups shredded cheddar

1/2 cup salsa of choice

12 medium flour tortillas

 Garden egg sliced or chopped.

Cooking Instruction;

Slice and chop your veggies, and rinse and drain the beans.

Heat olive oil in a large skillet over medium heat until shimmering.

Add onion and saute for 2 minutes,
stirring occasionally. Stir in garlic
and saute just briefly before adding
in the mushrooms.

Cook mushrooms over medium
heat, stirring occasionally, for about
7 minutes or until they have
softened and started to brown.

at the end of the mushroom's
cooking time, heat a separate
skillet over medium heat.

 Heat tortillas by ones or twos on
each side until lightly browned and
more pliable, then remove them to
a separate plate for filling.

After you have sauteed your mushrooms, stir in the pumpkin leaves and continue to cook over medium heat just until wilted and bright green.

Stir in the black beans and spices and heat.

Reduce heat under the pan to low. Stir in cheese until melted, then stir in salsa.

Divide the black bean/mushroom filling evenly among the tortillas and roll them up into burritos, fill or top with garden chopped and fresh sliced cucumbers.

BAKED CUCUMBER AND PUMPKIN WITH YOGHURT DRESSING AND HONEY FILLING:

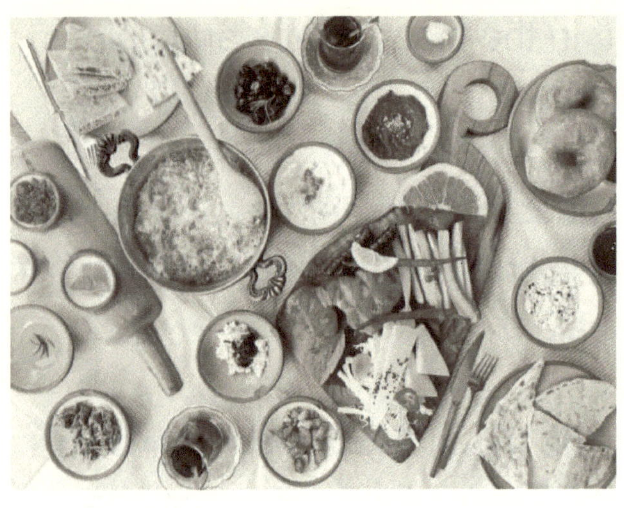

Ingredients:

2 medium sized cucumber

3-4 tablespoon of honey

1 cup coconut milk

2-3 full avocado

½ cup liquid milk

1teaspoon of sugar to taste

⅓ cup soya bean (powdered/or about 3 tablespoon) this is optional

Apple Cider vinegar (taste to know when enough)

Instruction:

Peel out avocados, and remove the entire fruit,blend together with liquid milk,sugar, soyabean and apple cider until smooth enough

Pour in the coconut milk and blend together you should make it thick .

/2 cup unsweetened natural flavored coconut yogurt

To get your pumpkin chips,follow this method:

Preheat the oven to 220°F. Line 2 baking sheets with parchment paper. ...

If desired, cut circle shapes with a biscuit cutter or cookie cutter. …

Roll the cut pumpkins with salt and pepper (if you like Pepper) for taste and dipped in honey preferably for a unique taste!

Bake for about 20-25 minutes
Don't leave it to get too crispy,just have it a bit soft

Slice cucumbers into a bit large sizes

To make the raspberry coulis for the filling: Put the raspberries and 1 tbsp icing sugar into the bowl of a food processor and blend to a purée adding enough honey ,thick enough...

Set a sieve over a clean bowl and rub the purée through to remove the raspberry pips.

To serve, whisk the cream and remaining icing sugar until softly peaked. Swirl in the raspberry coulis. Spoon or pipe the honey cream onto half the pumpkin and sandwich with the remaining pumpkins while dipping the cucumbers in-between

EGG TOMATO AND CUCUMBER SLICE:

Ingredients:
Enough circular sliced tomatoes
Enough thin sliced cucumber
3-4 eggs
2 tablespoon of honey
1 teaspoon olive oil

Instruction;

Slice tomatoes and cucumbers,whisk eggs,add onions , Pepper,salt to taste and olive oil and add honey.

Pour your egg into a microwave safe oven container or bowl,add the sliced tomato and cucumbers and heat in the oven for a few Minutes.

Serve bread, perfect for breakfast!

FRIED VEGGIE MELON SAUCE:

Ingredients:

Grinded melon seeds (powdered)
Osu
Crayfish
Pepper
Meat
Black fish
Stockfish
Periwinkle
Palm oil
Onions
Vegetables
Seasonings
Ginger
Garlic

Cooking Instruction;

Cook meat and stockfish with onions seasoning with a little salt, once it's almost ready add black fish and periwinkles,

   allow to cook a little, bring it down and set aside. Why you added the blackfish later is to avoid it from scattering too much.

Put oil in a dry pot and allow to heat up a little
Add your onions and fry for a sec.

Get a bowl, add your melon seeds powdered (is usually dried before

grinded) pepper, crayfish, osu and seasonings.
 Add little water to mix everything thoroughly.
Scoop the mixture in the hot oil and start frying it constantly to avoid it burning.

Once the grinded melon looks like crumbs then it's ready.

Add ur stock with the meat and all the rest u have set aside. If d stock water is small den add little water and just cover it.

It will cake on its own then you can turn it and check d thickness if it's ok by you or you still wanna add little water.

Then   add vegetable or bitterleaf, waterleave is the best for it, you can also use spinach or broccoli, depending on your choice.

Serve with made millet,or any soup food

CHICKEN LETTUCE WRAPS:

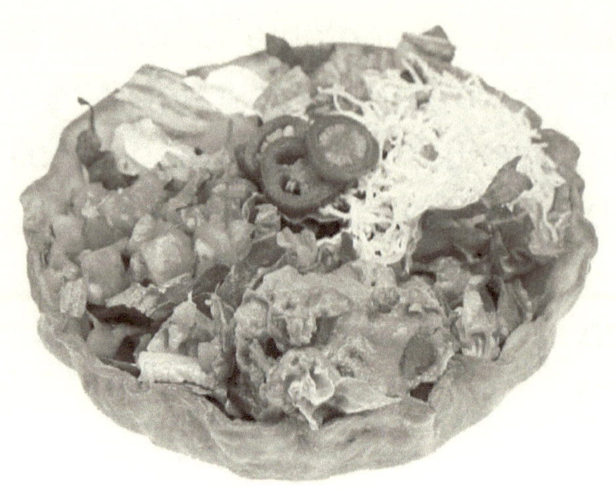

Ingredients:

2 Cups Of flour

1 tablespoon olive oil(vegetable oil)

⅓ teaspoon of salt

2 chicken breast

½ lime juice

⅓ teaspoon red chili pepper

1 teaspoon garlic powder

4 tablespoon of Groundnut oil

Lettuce

2-3 tomato

1-2 Onions

Mayonnaise/cream

 3-4 eggs

5-6 thin carrots (chopped)

Instruction;

 For the dough:

2 cups plain flour. 1 cup warm water. 1tablespoon of oil.1/3teaspoon salt. Mix everything together in a clean bowl. Knead it with a few drops of oil allow it to rest for 15 mins. Cover with nylon.

2. Get 2 chicken breasts cut in strips. To marinate the chicken:

Add 1tsp of salt. 1/2 Lime juice. 1/3 tsp red chilli powder. 1tsp garlic powder.

You can also use the fresh one. 4tablespoon of . Oil in a clean bowl. Add the shredded chicken. Cover & allow to rest for 1hr. 3. Bring out the dough.

Sprinkle flour on your table. Make 5 dough balls. Make it flat like rolling meat pie.

Rub in melted butter & roll it in. Put them in nylon, leave for five minutes & roll it out round very thin flat.

Spread them in a tray separately. Heat your non - stick pan or frying pan. Add 1 Tbs of g.oil, put the rolled out dough away for 1min & turn the other side.
Pour in a handful of carrots to every dough

Add 1 tbS of g. Oil again allow for 1 minute. Do the same for all. 4. In a clean bowl or plate add 1 cup of flour.

1/4 tsp of chilli powder. 1/3 of salt. Mix very well. Break one egg in another small plate.

Heat oil for frying. Deep the marinated chicken inside the egg and pour in the remaining carrots,(you should have enough carrots for this) and dust it inside the dried flour mixture & fry until golden brown.

Remove & put it in a serveth or clean towel not to soak oil. 5. Wash & Cut 2 - 3 tomatoes as you want. 1 onion. Don't slice the Lettuce ,

You can just share it into two or 3. Make sure it is properly washed.

Bring out your wrap, put 2-3 of your fried chicken in the middle, arrange the sliced onions and tomatoes, add the lettuce.

Then add your mayonnaise or cream as you like but not much .

VEGETABLE SOUP:

spinach

Waterleaf

Meat any type of your choice

Stockfish

Black fish

Periwinkle with the shell or without

d shell ur choice.

Crayfish

Fresh red bell pepper or yellow bell

pepper .

Palm oil

Onions

Mushrooms

(Use ingredients depending on the

quantity you want to make)

Cooking Instruction;

Wash meat and stock fish with salted water.

Cook with little water and add onions and seasonings with a pinch of salt.

be very careful with putting salt, vegetable and salt are enemies. Practically….

Once it's almost done, wash ur black fish with hot water and add to it along with periwinkle without shell. Allow to steam for few 5mins

While meat is cooking thoroughly wash the vegetables with salt

in your boiling meat add crayfish and pepper mix well and add palm oil /(any other oil you have)and allow to cook together with meat.

The oil has to be cooked well too to give the taste you want.
Add waterleaf and turn together after turning it, also add ur

vegetables and mushrooms, and turn all together.

Check for the taste if there is a need to correct seasoning, add.

Add onions lastly and cover for a few seconds and bring it down to maintain the greenish and freshness of the vegetable.

Your soup is ready to be eaten with, semo, or wheat.
Your choice!

HONEY-Lemon MANGO JAM:

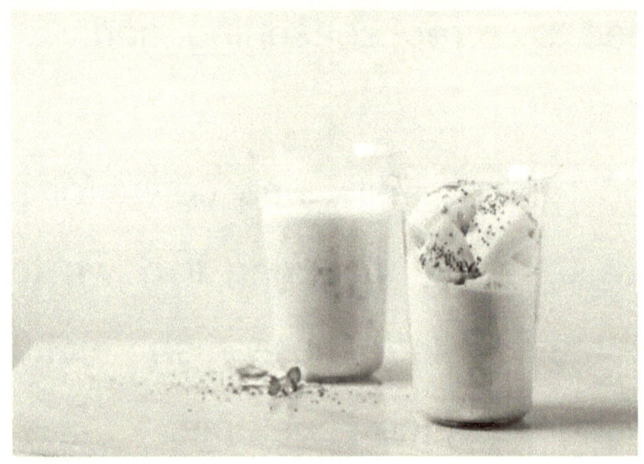

Ingredients:

•2 cup of mangoes

•50g of sugar

1-2 Tablespoons of lemon

2-3 tablespoon of honey

1 handful of almond

¼ cup almond milk

1 teaspoon apple cider vinegar

Instruction;

Cut the mango pieces first and blend

Put the mixture into a bowl and add the sugar and lemon and other ingredients

Heat for some minutes, stirring well to combine

Keep it tight and pack in

Freeze.

VEGGIE CARROTS AND EGG BEANS MEAL:

Ingredients:

3 cups of Beans ,

2 Onions,

1 teaspoon Thyme,

1-2 teaspoon curry,

½ Ginger,

1 clove of Garlic ,

crayfish ,

1 medium sized Tomatoes (sliced),

 Red Fresh pepper ,

Red chili pepper

2-3 eggs ,

Roasted fish

salt to taste

6-7 thin carrots (or big ones,

anyhow you like it!)

groundnut oil.

1st step :

Remove the back of the beans

depend on the quantities you want

to use(you soak it in water for

some Minutes and use your hand

to rub off the coat peels

Note;not all beans can be used,you can check for smaller size beans (seeds)

2nd step:
add all the ingredients except curry & groundnut oil before grinding it(blending the beans and Ingredients together,don't cook the beans before blending or grinding)

3rd step:
    put oil on the fry pan ,not too much oil, add small slice Onions & curry for 5minutes , U sieve it

and pour only the oils into the grinded beans ,it should be a kind of thick

.4th step: mix it very well ,add ur smoke fish ,& salt and extra seasoning,if any stir well to get the whole taste . Pour in your carrots chopped vegetables (cabbage, spinach,etc)

Place your pot on the fire ,add little water in the pot, pour in the whole dough either on aluminium foils or waterproof nylons or closeable portable plates , leave for about 50 minutes or ,1 hr

.

Serve! Enjoy!

PUMPKIN AND PEPPERED CRAB WITH AVOCADO:

Ingredients ;

Pumpkin

Avocado

Crab

Fresh crayfish

Scent leaf

Yellow pepper

Dry crayfish

Onion

Maggi & salt

Pepper soup spice

Water

Cooking Instruction;

Put your washed crab in a pot add onion, maggi ,salt little dry pepper & quantity of water you want to use for the soup
allow to boil after 20min add your washed fresh crayfish pounded

yellow pepper & grounded dry crayfish add little salt and maggi if need be

After 5min add your pepper soup spice stare and leave it to boil for another 5min then add your scent leaf after

Add chopped broccoli

After 3 Minutes take if off heat

Cook pumpkins with salt and any other ingredients you want

Serve crab Peppered soup with cooked pumpkin and top or place as side sliced avocados.

OVEN BAKED VEGGIE AND FRUITS PIE:

Filling:

Minced garlic

Onions

Carrots

Frozen peas

Irish potatoes (chopped)

Salt

Seasoning

Thyme

Black pepper

Scotch Bonnet

White pepper

Cabbage-chopped

Spinach-chopped

Spirulina leaves -chopped

Almond leaves-chopped

Cucumbers -sliced

Mayonnaise-cream

Lemon-sliced

Apple-sliced

Avocado pear sliced

Dough:

6 cups of Flour

4 Tbsp of White sugar

1 Tbsp of Baking powder

1 Tbsp of Salt

500grms of Cold butter

Evaporated Milk

4 Eggs

Instruction;

Saute onions in a pan till they are translucent, add mince garlic saute.

Add all seasonings and salt,cooked diced potatoes,carrots and peas.

Add your chopped vegetables,

Cook for like 8-10mins.

Remove from heat and allow to cool.

Add butter to dry ingredients (flour salt baking powder) and break up until it looks like a cornmeal.

Add wet ingredients (milk and eggs) and knead.

Transfer to a floured surface and knead until the dough is "fine".

Cut out shapes of the pie you want with any cutter of your choice e.g tea cup saucer.

Add filling, and dress with cream inside or Mayonnaise

close and press the sides down
with a fork.

Bake for 40-60mins in a preheated
350° oven

Enjoy! Your veggie pie!

PEANUT FRUIT BUNS:

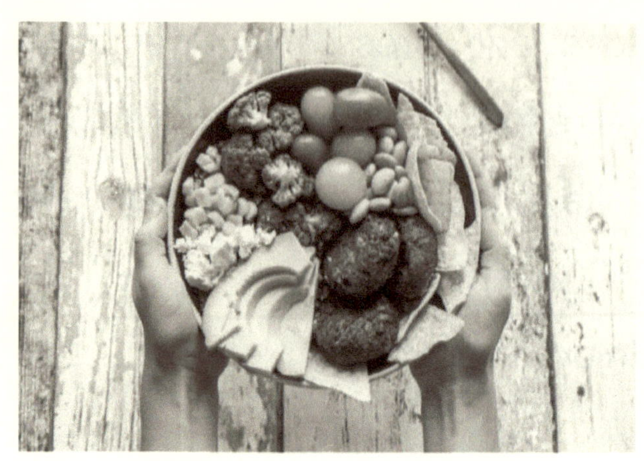

Ingredients;

Peanut

Flour 1kg

Yeast 24g

milk/water 600ml apx

Eggs 4-6 pcs

Butter/margarine 250g

Castro sugar 120g

Mixed fruit,

sultana, mixed chopped peel(grate the back of orange and lemon)-300g

Currant, mixed chopped peel

Instruction;

Add your flour in a mixing bowl

Add your butter

Add yeast, eggs, sugar, pinch of salt and mix thoroughly and allow to rest

Brush the dough with egg after using the rolling pin to flatten it.

After brushing it with egg, pour icing sugar on the dough

Add mixed fruits and roll, cut with a knife (desired shape). Stuff with peanut

Then Place it in the oven till is done

VEGGIE CHICKEN CURRY SAUCE:

Ingredients:

1. Vegetable oil

2. Onions

3. Mixed Veggies (Carrot, green peas, green beans, yellow pepper, green pepper, red pepper.

4. Spices(curry, thyme, cubes, salt)

5. Ginger

6. Flour(for thickening if desired)

7. Chicken portions

Cooking Instruction:

---Firstly, steam your Chicken with spices to taste,
add onions and ginger, for flavour and chopped scotch bonnet as much as you can tolerate. Add

some water and allow it to cook
until quite soft.

--Hit up your vegetable oil in a
different pan as you would when
making stew.
Add a pinch of salt, then the sliced
or chopped onions depending on
how you prefer it. Then bit by bit,
layer by layer, start to add the
veggies...allowing them to cook
before adding more. Stir gently.

--Add the Chicken portions and stir.
 Allow to cook for 5minutes before
you add the stock. Stir gently.
Sprinkle some curry for colour,
cubes,and salt to taste. Stir and
allow to boil.

--if not as thick as you would want, mix a little flour with water and add to your sauce. Stir well. Allow to cook for another 3-5 minutes.

Tada! Ready to serve!

CARROT POTATO BREAD ROLLS:

Ingredients:-

 2 Irish potatoes,

3 finger carrots,

Green pepper(quantity to your taste)

A handful of green bean,

1 ginger, garlic,

A teaspoon of salt and cubes to taste,

black/ red pepper,

fish oil.

Bread.

Procedure:-

--Add grated potatoes, carrots, diced green bean, pepper, red pepper, ginger, garlic, salt, black pepper, and taste cubes and stir fry in fish oil for 2minutesand set aside.....

--pour in whisked raw egg (2) and stir......
Roll bread with a rolling pin on a chop board until flat and cut out the edges....

--add a spoonful of ur stir fried veggies on the rolled bread, brush water on the sides and roll and stick together at the edges...
Fry in a hot deep oil until golden brown.....

Serve with anything! Could be a smoothie or fruit juice!

HERBED TOMATO AND EGG FRY:

A delicious tomato and egg recipe!
Eggs cooked in a palate of herbs
and spices along with tomatoes,
served with a generous garnish of
fresh parsley!

Ingredients

30 Ml Olive oil
80 Gram Onion
10 Gram Garlic, chopped
1 Kg Ripe tomato
60 Gram Tomato paste
8 Gram Smoked paprika powder

8 Gram Cumin powder
5 Gram Cayenne pepper powder
10 Gram Salt
5 Gram Dried herbs
6 Nos Eggs
10 Gram Parsley, chopped

Cooking Instruction:

Heat olive oil in a large lidded

frying pan over a medium heat and

add the onion. Cook until golden

and then add peppers.

Add garlic and dried herbs and
cook for another couple of minutes.
Pour in the tomatoes and roughly
mash.

Stir the mixture and bring to a boil, then turn down the heat and simmer.
Add all remaining spices and seasoning and cook on low heat for 15 minutes.
Make 4-8 divots in the sauce and

break in the eggs.

Season them lightly, turn the heat

right down as low as possible,

cover and cook for about 10

minutes until they're just set.

Serve with fresh chopped parsley.

(Pictures were removed to match publishing standards)

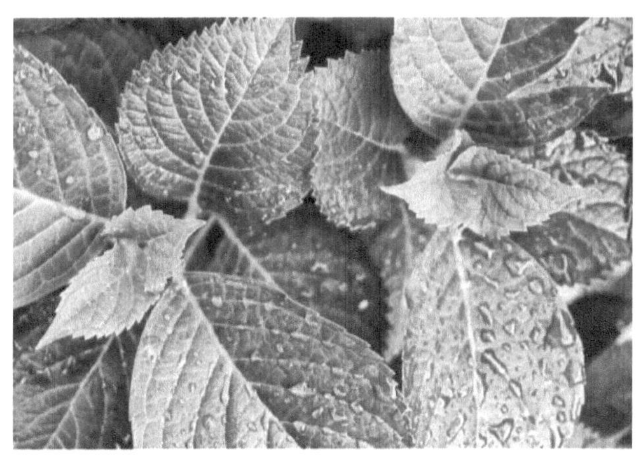

CHAPTER 2:

16 MEDICINAL FOODS AND THEIR HEALTH BENEFITS+CURATIVE PROPERTY:

LEMON GRASS:

Lemon grass is an antibacterial and can be used as a treatment to most bacterial infections and caused diseases,
Lemon grass is a good body activator and helps in the smooth running of the blood system, including the whole body system,...

Perfect for the immune system,it boosts it very well , giving the body defensive antibodies and agents against diseases and sickness,which is ,in essence there's a reduced risk of being prone to diseases.
It can be used for the treatment of typhoid,
Fever,

Malaria fever,
Typhoid fever,
Purging, stooling and vomiting
Stomach upset and more

……

AVOCADO PEAR:

the persea Americana is not
just a wonderful fruit to be eating
as food but also one of mother
nature's medicinal fruits ,used as
treatment to various sickness,in
various ways,which includes using
the seed , cutting it into different
parts and soaking it in water for a
few days,which is a good treatment
and remedy for peptic ulcer,
moreover this method has proven

to be one of the good ways in chasing peptic ulcer if taken consistently,with the right dosage,is also good to note that this apparatus doesn't work for all….

Why?..
Because all people on earth have different body systems,while some body systems,could be very open and responsive to the usage of some natural remedies,some wouldn't and that's just how it works,so if it works for you Great! If it doesn't,well you have to stop the medication (if you're using it as a remedy to a sickness)

It also has a hard knock against Malaria,

Gastrointestinal problems and
insomnia,
Hypertension and also is good for
getting your hair all nice and
healthy!

COCONUT:

   the Cocos nucifera is good for
the immune system,it also helps to
fighting against some ailments,its
water is used to stop hangover
haha ,Incase you didn't know when
you drink a lot to stupur , coconut
water gets you hydrated and back
to life,
The water is also used to stop
reactions by drugs when taken

wrongly or overdosage, the water is blessed with life! And is a very good antioxidant

A Boost in Good Cholesterol. ...
Good for Blood Sugar and Diabetes. ...
Helps Fight Back Against Alzheimer's Disease. ...
Helps Stop Heart Disease and High Blood Pressure. ...
Aids in Liver Health. ...
Boosts Energy. ...
Aids with Digestion.
And for the men,Good news! Coconut water is very good for your "men's health" it boosts your sperm count and boosts your potency..in other words it makes you stronger !

The other parts of the plant can be
used for treatment to various
illnesses including,
bronchitis,fibroid,toothache,dysente
ry and Even toothache,the water is
known to be an anti poison!

APPLE:

This beautiful fruit is known not
just to give tonnes of vitamins and
minerals but also an antibiotic
It also gives a boost to the
immune system for proper
mechanism….the red local apple
should contain more of these
goodies!

Apple contains pectin,a soluble
fibre that can lower high blood
pressure, reducing the risk of heart
diseases
If you're having constant pain in the
waist be sure to constantly
consume apples,
It aids in calming constipation,
Also treatment for diarrhea

PLANTAGO MAJOR:

Different from the plantain which
we all commonly know,in my
opinion,I think this plant is mainly
for sexual health,like this is its
base,like every other plants and
fruits has a speciality also.

Extracted cold extract from the plant fruit makes sperm real thick and also increases sperm count, maintaining its antibacterial properties.

So for those who struggle and fight with bacterial infections,maybe exposure to public toilets or other high prone means of contacting infections, should think of using these natural antibacterial fruits and plants because it will definitely have a effect after, and please be sure to get proper guidelines before self medicating especially with natural ingredients, because they are really strong medicines, and please while taking any natural remedies be sure not to engage in drugs , because the two can't and won't work together

…(Incase you will ever need guidance on any of the natural remedies which will be discussed at the finale of this book,my socials are always open! And I'm always available to help you!)

It is rich in potassium, mucilage and zinc, including flavonoid, it is also used to combat inflammation of the mucus membrane.

MISTLETOE:

While many love using this beautiful all purpose herb to cook food it can also be an excellent herb against some certain sickness.

Those who eat mistletoe are protected and has a low chance of getting cancer

Mistletoe grows on a tree where the tree gets cancer….
It also helps in treating cancer,if you have cancer you can be constantly using it to cook,or just boil it and eat it like a snack !

It also contains alkaloids, useful in problems associated with gynecology, stroke,cancer and even hypertension,
Obviously for the elderlies more, elderlies should consume more of natural foods, vegetables and fruits

234

including known herbs as it makes them stronger and still fresh looking

Who wouldn't love to have a Granny or pa who is so healthy and strong?!
Well, vegetables and fruits is the answer, some herbs work more than some drugs…..an apple a day gets the doctor away,isn't it? ,But nevertheless take drugs when necessary!

EUPHORBIA HIRTA:

Hey….. are you with me???

Don't worry about the name,is not some kind of ancient mysterious herb you probably never heard of ...well is still mysterious though..

We are talking about Asthma weed,yes ! That's it
It is a herbal plant for asthmatic patients,like I said our body systems are all different what cures your neighbor may not cure you or prove useful to your desired result, nevertheless it helps,not minding the body system, simply because of its abilities and properties

The leave is usually dried to be taken and mostly used for treatments or infusion…

Talking of herbal wonders, this is good in combating dysentery, bronchitis, hypertension, constipation etc ,if not permanently stopping it…

Good news again for men and women alike,it increases libido , yeah that's Right,and in women it increases lactations and…….shape of breast!

How come vegetarians,are so strong,fit,in perfect shape,and so healthy and hot probably? Well mother nature gave us a great gift didn't she?

Embrace nature!

BITTER LEAF:

bitter leave is known,as the name implies for its extreme bitterness,but my friend this is one of the few plants that helps the liver and kidney to function properly,
It filters the kidney, flushing out every bacteria and diseases present,

It Is very good in stopping stomach upset or any form of pain in the abdomen, including frequent stooling with a quick response!
It is a cathartic that makes you purge out all the bad stuff in your system, giving your intestines a thorough clean!

Be ready to be visiting the white house in your home…

Also used in the treatment of arthritis, insomnia, prostrate cancer,gonorrhea and loss of memory
  And it is used as a stopper to stop blood flowing from wounds and/or cuts it heals and concedes fast…
The leave is usually washed with hands , just like washing a cloth and scrumbling it ,like 4 times before drinking or is gonna be too bitter for you

GARLIC:

Well who doesn't know garlic and it's health benefits? ,
The allium sativum is one of the oldest known natural antibiotics, usually used as food,for spicing and seasoning.

It is an antifungal,anticancer ,antiviral,and anti-parasitic, it is a great immune booster, it releases allicin that reduces inflammation in the body. This acts as an antioxidant, reducing damage from free radicals to the body's cells that contribute to the disease.

 garlic can help stimulate circulation and blood flow to sexual organs in both men and women. However, because of garlic's smell,do not eat often or sure when

you know you won't be meeting
many people (haha)
It may also reduce the risk of
common brain diseases like
Alzheimer's disease and dementia,
it contains antioxidants that protect
against cell damage and aging,

It can be used in the treatment of
fever, Asthma,cough,and
Ringworm etc.

CHICKWEED:

The larrea tridentate is said to
contain a possible great amount of
antioxidants, preventing the body
from certain cancers and diseases.

It can be used in the treatment of fracture,ulcer and many skin diseases

CORN:

the zea maize is a good source of carbohydrate as we all know, but there's a very remarkable thing about corn and some certain things it could do with a simple paratus

Incase of kidney stone,or cancer ,get corn silk and boil it , drink it as you drink your coffee,it will help to cure,and one more marvel! If you're looking to lose some weight,this could be good too as it also helps in curing obesity

SCENT LEAF:(ñchánwû)

The scent lea is a good natural spice and seasoning, mostly for cooking pepper soups,fish,meats and even foods like rice
It has the ability of changing the food's aroma and taste, when used for pepper soup it adds to its use .

It contains antibodies and also a good antibiotic,for someone who eats a lot of pastries or already made foods you should start adding some of this natural spice as they reduce and entice this junkies bad effect on our Health

It is used to stop stomach
pains,and stomach upsets.

PIGEON PEAS:

pigeon peas is a blood tonic
and booster, it is used in the
treatment of sickle cell anaemia,
Kidney purifier,
Also used by persons who suffered
severe loss of blood following a
long period of ailment

CARROT:

the daucus carota is Identified to contain a high amount of carotene, carotene prevents cancer and eye defects,

   Carotene aids in digestion and Lower's Cholesterol.
  Good news for Men
Carrot eaten with Groundnut promotes thickness of the sperm.

Including Cotton leaves
Which is also good for blood

MUSTARD SEED:

In a nutshell,this is a miracle seed,one of the oldest and greatest most effective anti poison I have ever come across to

If you feel like you have eaten
something or taken in something to
your body system that doesn't
seem right , mustard seed makes
you alright!
Is a miracle seed

CHAPTER 3:

8 TOP VITAMINS WITH LONGEVITY PROPERTIES:

NIACIN:

Vitamin B3 is one of the top vitamins offering Longevity and healthy Lifestyle Milk,spirulina, chicken,breast milk,nuts and more are all good sources of Niacin

- Niacin helps in the production of insulin.

- It promotes and aids in sperm and ovaries production and maintenance.

- It Aide's in promoting better circulatory system

- Niacin helps in maintaining good and healthy skin

- Good for weight loss

- It aids digestion

PANTOTHENIC ACID:

Grains, spirulina,orange,egg,
pineapple are good sources of
vitamin B5

- It congeles blood when there's
  an injury,and it fasten the
  healing of injuries

- It boosts the immune system
  giving promotion to long life

- It supports growth

- It gives the body antibodies
  and defence against diseases

- Reduction of stress

- It acts as a mechanism to different glands In the body

COBALAMIN:

fish, spirulina,eggs milk,beans etc ,are all good sources of cobalamin

- It helps in the production of energy in our body

- It supports the brain,develops and improves it.

- Helps in combating fatigue and anaemia

- It encourages and support the formation of Healthy nerves and growth

- It Aide's in the multiplication and formation of cells

- It works alongside other vitamins and antibodies to function properly.

FOLIC ACID:

Folic acid can be found in milk, spinach, spirulina,and most green leaves!

- Folic acid is a brain's-essential;it is necessary for the proper working of neurotransmitter and the brain

- It stimulates appetite;it is a good "appetizer" it supports in the proper functioning of the liver

- It supports the vitamin B12 to produce healthy red blood cells.

- Very essential for pregnant women,for proper development

- Treats and prevent anemia

- It aid's in the production of protein nutrients the body needs,by working alongside other vitamins.

MAGNESIUM:

magnesium is a mineral which can be gotten from the consumption of natural foods and spices including, but not limited to, garlic, almond, onion, Lemon,and spirulina…

- Magnesium increases enzymic activities during metabolic processes for the production of energy in the brain,heart and within many other different organs in the body.

- Magnesium helps in the building of strong bones, conducting impulses in the nerve and the contraction of muscles.

- Magnesium as a helping mineral, works alongside phosphorus and calcium.

- Magnesium helps to strengthen the heart and blood vessels against the development of possible diseases and problems of the heart.

- Magnesium has also proven in some way to be an enzyme,With the fact it helps to convert sugars in the blood into Energy.

VITAMIN C:

Although vitamin c is common,and almost found in all

citric fruits,it is one of the best vitamin, giving Longevity to the human body and a magnificent boost to the immune system.

Vitamin c is gotten from fruits like orange which has a significant high amount of the vitamin in it, Lemon,grape,guava,apple, banana,pawpaw, spirulina and more….

- Vitamin c has proven to be the best antioxidant

- It shields the body against infections

- Taking a high dose of vitamin c prevent and chase away

Candida, bacterium,and degenerative ailments.

- Vitamin c strengthens the body tissues

- Vitamin c helps in keeping protein collagen

- Vitamin c has an anti ageing agent which helps in the prevention of premature ageing

- Vitamin c helps in the healing of injury and protects the body from radical damage

- For people looking to lose weight vitamin c decreases cholesterol and repairs cell

ZINC:

Zinc is an essential vitamin/mineral needed in our body systems, however it can be gotten from the consumption of mushrooms, spirulina (this has many vitamins and minerals it gives) and sunflower extracts.

- Zinc gives an agent which helps fastening the rate at which wounds and burns heal

- Zinc is needed in the body for the production of hormones

- Zinc supports and promotes healthy reproduction systems in male and female.

- Zinc is also used medically for prevention and healing of most prostate problems

- Zinc is also good for the males as it helps boost Healthy sperm production and produces insulin.

- It supports male and female fertility and also increases the senses of smell and vision

- Zinc promotes healthy skin and a booster to the immune system to fight infections.

SELENIUM:

Selenium is an antioxidant which works well with the vitamin E, Spirulina is mostly found in grains, and also spirulina the all round veggie

- Selenium contains an anti ageing property

- Selenium helps in fighting heart diseases and cancer

- It supports growth and fertility

- Selenium is also required by the body for the essential utilisation of fatty acids,and helps in fighting inflammation.

- It promotes the production of glands , including   the prostaglandins

CHAPTER 4:

(SPECIAL)RECIPES FOR LIFE:stay positive!!;

1.

The recipe for happiness!

Hello! For the recipe of happiness you need these six **ingredients** below:

3 Handfuls of **generosity**

3 full cups of **patience**

1 heartful of **kindness**

1 full headful of **Understanding**

3 tablespoons of **goodness**

1 heartful of **love**

1 soulful of **faith**

Instruction:

Mix goodness ,   patience
and understanding, sprinkle
With Love,
and serve with generosity!

Serving:

with all through a lifetime!
Serve with everyone you
Meet.

2.

PATIENCE:A formula!

Practice great   **P**atience with all

Seek to develop **A**bilities

Value your   **T**ime always

Take the   **I**nitiative in work

Follow Master's **E**xample

Put aside   **N**on life essential

Cultivate a good **C**haracter

Never fail to put in **E**fforts no

Matter failure.

3.

13 key ingredients To Remember !

Never fail to remember **THE....**

Virtue of   **effort**

Worth of **Sacrifices**

Love   of **Contentment**

Effectiveness of **Concentration**

Dignity of **Simplicity**

Value   of **Time**

Virtue   of **patience**

Peace of **Trust**

Importance of **Positivity**

Power   of **Love**

Model   of   **Good example**

Joy   of   **Charity**

Fulfilled heart of **kindness**

4.

8 Elements To live by!

Share the **love** to live by

Practice the **Charity** to live by

Show **mercy** to live by

Utilize the **happiness** to live by

Develop the **faith** to live by

Cultivate the **courage** to live by

Hunger for **success** to live by

The power of **knowledge** to live by

5

*Reach out to Your
Desired Recipe And Enjoy!*

Now have a seat,Get your pot of concentration ready,make ready your best ingredients To achieve that goal and enjoy!

Now this is all you need to get your desired recipe and be filled!

Firstly,free your mind from depression, anxiety, worry,sadness and negativity and any other elements that can give your food a bad taste,
Now fill that mind with positive thought,and keep stirring with Positivity.

Free your heart ,free it from hatred and any impurity there, remember you wouldn't be a good cook if you keep dirtying your white ……,if your ingredient bag is heavy and loaded with all sorts of leftovers and rubbish,that can make your food taste bitter, how would you find the right ingredients needed to get to your recipe's highest peak and highest level of enjoyment and self fulfillment?

Now fill it with love! Yeah that's great! Way to Go!!

Now,live simply and in contentment,didn't get the right taste for the recipe? Oh don't worry you still can try again! Yes try again,and know that you did absolutely great for trying,be happy , keep it simple and be content with your little result, nevertheless next time trying it ,put in Efforts and more   concentration   and consideration!

Do not expect much though,forget the pronouns "SELF" "I" , think more of the "YOU" "OTHERS" come on,you can seek advice from someone else who knows better than you,let down pride if there's any,and don't forget....be sure to also care for others too, you can invite them for a meal!

   now we are about done.Do to others what you would have others do for you!

In pursuit of a goal and happiness,use this recipe!

6.

Apply The Great Ingredient: LOVE!

Haaaaa who doesn't have this great ingredient ? ,You don't have it? Well sorry to disappoint you but we all have that great ingredient,we all have that one essential and a must! Even infants do!,

Yeah, unless you don't want to use your great ingredient for a great taste ,unless you are hiding it, maybe from past experience,or whatever it be the reason you are not using it,I want you to let go! Yes ! Let it go.

Nothing is worth You not using your great ingredient for great dishes! You're missing a lot if you think that way, but don't worry let's get that ingredient, develop it and start using it because it is important as life itself,shall we? ….I hear you say   YES!

Love is the only good,the only light and the only gold needed for a great tasty life!

Love to man is like honey to bees

Love sees no obstacles or barriers,no limits!

Love is a natural Ingredient with its willingness to protect, preserve and sacrifice!

Love is the force driven to life success and happiness

Love a mysterious energy and ingredient no man can do without

Love cares for others well being as well as self

Love grows with you day in day out!

Love is the magnificent divinity in you! It is your speciality!

Love is a wonder and a joy to the soul and mind

Love trust's and understands

Love is always positive,it feels your home and life fresh with positivity!

Love fears not and hate's not

Love is happy with the success and life of others!

7.

First, Create A Picture Of Your Desired Delicacy In Mind!

Well all you have to do here is **Think** it first then act on it,work to it and strive for it

*Success can come your way anytime anyday all you have to do is **think it! Create a picture!***

*You can do and achieve all the goals you have set for yourself and execute plans! All you have to do is **think it ! Create a picture!***

*Before you do things, before you take actions, first of all **Think it! Create a picture!***

Think** that you may rise up so high and get the bigger prize! Think **it! Create a picture

*You have to be positive all the time,all you have to do is **think it** and **create a picture***

Think** how you can give out to many people,donate to charities,share your love and other valuables and help people in utmost need and bring joy to each and everyone you come across to,is **possible** all you have to do is **think it** and **create a picture!.

8.

Avoid Getting Yourself Spilled With Dirt!

In the course of duty here in life,there are some certain things to avoid,and guess what? They seem to give bad and negative energies!

So avoid them!

*If you are always covered with **pride,** you will always be thrown aside and matched to the ground.*

*One who is filled with **hate** will forever be in a bad state*

*One who enjoys **deceit** and it's council will get hit in one way or another and it will be a huge blow*

*One will never achieve transcendence, if they are dulled and clouded with **ignorance***

*They will never progress,they that find pleasure in **criticism***

*They that are always overshadowed by **negativity** will not see the light*

*One who is always troubled by **sadness** will be in constant misery*

*They that are easily overcomed by **fear** will remain in the dark*

***Jealousy** brings sorrow and self degradation*

*They that are clouded by **impossible illusions** will remain stagnant.*

9.

Enjoy   With   Your C.O.M.P.A.N.I.O.N!

Always use this self declaration when reaching out to people! Is important that you be selfless! It brings joy and peace of the mind soul,declare daily to yourself,make it a daily meal

Use this ingredient **COMPANION**

Now Say After Me!

I Shall………….

*...Show loving **C**are to people*

Utilize every   **O**pportunity to help

Show   **M**odesty always

Live   **P**olitely

Use my   **A**bility to serve

Serve the   **N**eeds of others

Noture   **I**ntegrity and honesty

Overcome all **O**bstacles

Develop immunity to **N**egativity!

10.

You can be.....
Successful *by learning from failure*

Healed *by letting go of the past!*

Great *by working towards greatness!*

Courageous *by defeating Fear*

Diligent *by putting a halt to laziness*

Declare with me.......

I must know what my goal is

I must be sure to want it

I must really be sure it is a good goal

I must believe I can reach my goal

I must cultivate positive thoughts

I must really strive towards reaching my goal and aims!

CHAPTER 5:

SPECIAL SECRET MIX FOR IMMUNE BOOSTER/FITNESS/HEALTHY CLEAN SYSTEM:

Okay this is a natural drink mix which heals and treats,and gives boost to immune system and defence against diseases,

If you take it enough and as often as possible you will notice Positive change in your body,this is also

great for weight loss,as it makes
you lighter and fit.

If you're looking to lose some
weight this can help you in the long
run,you don't have to read a 100
page book on weight loss before
you can lose weight, however it
requires a keen amount of effort.

However this solution is alcohol
Based ,and it helps in the
effectiveness of the medicine,
don't worry if you're not an alcohol
person you can use water you
don't have to worry because it
won't have bad implications on
your health

The core ingredient here is garlic,so first let's have a brief look on garlic:

Maximizing garlic's health benefits

The way garlic is processed or prepared can really change its health benefits.

The enzyme alliinase, which converts alliin into the beneficial allicin, only works under certain conditions. It can also be deactivated by heat.

One study found that as little as 60 seconds of microwaving or 45 minutes in the oven can deactivate alliinase and another study found similar results

However, it was noted that crushing garlic and allowing it to stand for 10 minutes before cooking can help prevent the loss of its medicinal properties.

The researchers also state that the loss of health benefits due to cooking could be compensated for by increasing the amount of garlic used.

Here are a few ways to maximize the health benefits of garlic:

Crush or slice all your garlic before you eat it. This increases the allicin content.

Before you cook with your crushed garlic, let it stand for 10 minutes.
Use a lot of garlic,more than one clove per meal, if you can

Recommended Garlic Intake daily:

The minimum effective dose for raw garlic is one segment (clove) eaten two to three times per day.

You can also take an aged garlic supplement. In that case, a normal dose is 600 to 1,200 mg per day.

High intakes of garlic supplements can be toxic, so don't exceed the dosage recommendations except if you know what you are doing.

Garlic is a strong immune booster:

Garlic contains compounds that help the immune system fight germs

Whole garlic contains a compound called alliin. When garlic is crushed or chewed, this compound turns into allicin (with a c), the main active ingredient in garlic

Allicin contains sulfur, which gives garlic its distinctive smell and taste.

However, allicin is unstable, so it quickly converts to other sulphur-containing compounds thought to give garlic its medicinal properties

These compounds have been shown to boost the disease-fighting response of some types of white blood cells in the body when they encounter viruses, such as the viruses that cause the common cold or flu

Now I am going to show you exactly what and how to mix the medicine

What's needed?

Don't worry, maybe your heart was probably pounding rocks haha "whoa is gonna be a hell lot of ingredients needed!can I get it all "

So,this is what is needed, depending on the quantity you want to make,but I'm suggesting, if you just want to test it to see how your body would react to it,then do it in a small quantity, when you're pleased with the results,you will know the quantity of ingredients to mix then!

All you need is Garlic,

Ginger,

Turmeric,

Lemon

And a diluted alcohol (not beer,but maybe Gin or any form of fresh alcohol that won't harm you)

You can use water to dilute too

The reason (s),for using alcohol is because this solution has proven to be the best ever and works more effectively

How to prepare:

Peel out the garlics,gingers,turmeric and lemon ,

Don't pound it or anything just cut it all into small sizes, put it together in a bottle or any container and pour in the alcohol, leave for at least 2,3-4 days to properly blend and condensed

Drink a short of it every morning, preferably a tumbler,
Please note: sometimes you have to skip days to avoid excess or overdosage,and have a break when possible.

It is a great immune booster and trust me if you're looking to lose weight you will testify after taking this,it makes you feel strengthened ,fit,and light!

About the taste?
Haha don't worry it tastes a little bit like alcohol and the other blended

ingredients, then you think you are an expert brewer

Pure honey has proven to be a great healer and an essential for our Health,add honey if you like.

If you don't go well with alcohol,dilute with water and let it ferment for 3 days….

I'm always available to help, questions and advice)

.

Here are five more ways to boost immune function and help you avoid colds and the flu:

- Eat a healthy, balanced diet: Your whole diet is important. Getting a balance of important nutrients will make sure your immune system stays in good shape.

- Take a zinc supplement: Take zinc lozenges or syrup within 24 hours of the start of a cold, as this may reduce the duration of the cold

- Take a probiotic: Probiotics can promote a healthy gut,

enhance your immune system and reduce your risk of infection

- Avoid excess alcohol: Excess alcohol is thought to damage your immune system and make you more susceptible to infections

- Don't smoke: Cigarette smoke can weaken your immune system and make you more prone to infection

kitchen tips:

To avoid tears while cutting onions. Before using the onion peel the back, put it in the fridge for 10mins, bring it out and use it.

Soak garlic in cold water for like a minute,and use your hand to remove the back ,it will come off easily.

To preserve beans from weevils and licks,remove dirt from beans and store in a jerry can with cover or put the beans in a nylon and get a bucket with cover.The beans will last and remain cool till the seed finishes.

Wrap your unused fresh vegetables inside a paper could be newspaper then keep cold.

When peeling banana or plantain apply oil in your hands so as to avoid the sticking.

Preserve your dry fish and crayfish inside the freezer with a tight closed container.

To cut pepper with bare hands ,apply vegetable oil on the hand and cut the pepper,the effect will not be felt

If you're boiling rice and it's too soft due to too much water just put a slice of bread on it and the bread will absorb the water and normalize the rice.

Incase hot water or hot oil mistakingly pour on any part of your body just pour flour on it immediately .... And your skin won't peel or swell up

Just a few garlic in the oil is used to fry chin chin or any other thing and the oil gets back fresh to be used for stew in case you don't have another. Add small lemon juice to your over salted soup, stew and it does magic.

Kitchen tips continued:

Prepare white soup,I.e cook the meat, keep it aside then boil stock fish, dry fish, salt, papper, crayfish, seasoning cube etc. Put it in the freezer, if none, add a little water and warm it every morning. Prepare with desired quantity of water then take the quantity as you want whenever you wanna prepare any kind of soup, even unripe plantain etc.

Note, don't put the meat in the white soup,it will be very very soft before the white soup will finish or you can cook it half done. Then as you warm it everyday, it gets soft .

When eating,and bone enters your throat cough and pull your ear at the same time it will be out!

Slice onions near fire to avoid watery eyes or Slice under water

Use cold water to melt small amounts of your Semo vita before adding your hot water this will make it free from lumps.

If your meat is small in shape, parboil for some seconds without water this will help to raise the meat then you can add water and seasoning.

Fry curry leaf together with tomatoes.. That stew will be the sweetest.

If you want to enjoy ice fish ,don't boil it.Just wash and marinate,when you are ready to fry,slice onions in the oil and fry.

To reuse already use oil, grate few ginger and fry for some seconds it will remove the odour or flavour of what you fried initially and taste fresh

To cook beans faster , after the first water drains, add chopped onions into it and add water.

Use eggshell or grounded garlic and salt to get rid of wall geckos

For a crunchy Irish potato , soak it in water (not salty water)at least 30 minutes before frying. For yam and sweet potato, soak overnight.

Make crayfish the last ingredient u add to every meal. The taste of the meal is WOW

To avoid getting your tomato burnt while preparing for a stew, frying tomato for stew, add dry pepper…

Do you know you can use raw beans to boil hard meat?

Always add slice tomatoes to your food it helps to reduce cholesterol

SECTION TWO

LOSE WEIGHT FAST WITHOUT MUCH HARD WORK

A Simple In-A-Nutshell ways to lose a considerable amount of weight without much hard work,

Featuring:

How not to gain weight
Simple daily routine plans
Exercise and meal plans
Watching your weight,
Laugh pills(Essential for burning calories)
Natural medicine for weight loss

……and lots more!

Table Of Contents:

CHAPTER ONE:

<u>BEST EXERCISES FOR WEIGHT LOSS</u>

CHAPTER SEVEN:

<u>WEIGHT LOSS AID DRINK</u>

CHAPTER EIGHT:

<u>LAUGH PILLS:A MEDICINE FOR WEIGHT LOSS</u>

CHAPTER ONE:

INTRODUCTION

Hi there welcome to the next section of this book,here you will be getting simple and quick easy ways to lose weight, you don't need a 50 or 100 page book to lose weight,what matters is the information contained,and it's vitality and impact it will have on you.

So,I am going to keep it as simple
as possible,I don't believe you
have to work your ass off before
you lose some weight, well
although it really involves some
level of commitment,and it really is
a journey.

I am more than happy that you
have decided to make an ultimate
choice concerning your body and
embarking on this journey,I just
want to let you know that you are
not alone!

You have taken the first necessary

step already,and I bet you won't be

giving up…..will you?? Oh I hear

you say "NO"! That's great to hear

then,let's proceed lovelies!

I am better off called Emscent,I
started a great journey 4 and a half
years ago,I am a fitness trainer and
philosopher by heart and nature,I
love nature and it loves me.

Haha never mind,I just want to let

you know right now I am light as a

bird ,and you too can! Although I

never was "weighty" but trust me I

weighed a lot when I was

"younger"

Now let's just get to the explanation
of weight before proceeding…..

nah it isn't going to be bored ,I
know you weren't expecting this ,
but chill…..

The Human Body Weight:

According to wik,Human body weight refers to a person's mass or weight. Body weight is measured in kilograms, a measure of mass, throughout the world.

although in some countries such as the United States it is measured in pounds, or as in the United Kingdom, stones and pounds. Most hospitals, even in the United States, now use kilograms for calculations, but use kilograms and pounds together for other purposes

body weight is the measurement of weight without items located on the person. Practically though, body weight may be measured with clothes on, but without shoes or heavy accessories such as mobile phones and wallets, and using manual or digital weighing scales.

 Excess or reduced body weight is regarded as an indicator of determining a person's health, with body volume measurement providing an extra dimension by calculating the distribution of body weight.

Weight in Children:

There are a number of methods to estimate weight in children for circumstances (such as emergencies) when actual weight cannot be measured. Most involve a parent or health care provider guessing the child's weight through weight-estimation formulas.

These formulas base their findings on the child's age and tape-based systems of weight estimation. Of the many formulas that have been used for estimating body weight, some include the APLS formula, the Leffler formula, and Theron formula.

There are also several types of tape-based systems for estimating children's weight, with the most well-known being the Broselow tape.

The Broselow tape is based on length with weight read from the appropriate color area. Newer systems, such as the PAWPER tape, make use of a simple two-step process to estimate weight: the length-based weight estimation is modified according to the child's body habitus to increase the accuracy of the final weight prediction.

The Leffler formula is used for children 0–10 years of age.In those less than a year old it is

and for those 1–10 years old it is

where m is the number of kilograms the child weighs and am and ay respectively are the number of months or years old the child is.

Credit: Wikipedia

Estimated weight around the world:

Hey?????

Are you with me? ,Now go back to that figure at the left row, yeah all those figures at the left row.....

Did you notice anything? That's to show you,tell you and explain to you that you are not alone in This,just look at the figures ,the numbers in percentage represents the total number of overweight/total population as you can see you're just a small member of something so much big

From the table,it clearly shows the countries with the population percentage of "weighty" people,so never feel mad or bad about your body! ,Well why would you? Not anymore, following my personal recommendations and guides ,

losing weight fast is sure ….ya dig?
I love you!

I have literally trained to the point I
can't finish a plate of food,well not
if the food is so sweet and
irresistible…. wouldn't you love it?
Having control over how much you
can eat ? Having control over your
weight and all? ….. stuff about to
change!!

CHAPTER TWO:

SIMPLE TIPS FOR WEIGHT LOSS:

I will be giving you simple and easy tips to losing weight,and you have to promise me one thing....just one thing

can you promise Yourself that you will not only read the contents of this book and then dump it afterwards? Can you promise yourself that you will effectively act on it to get your results?

Now Say this ,pledge to yourself,yes place your hand on your heart and say "*I WILL EFFECTIVELY TRY THE TIPS HEREIN,AND I WILL NEVER GIVE UP TILL I ACHIEVE MY GOAL!*" Say it once more ,this time with authority and determination,let's go!

Great!!! The initiation has been made ,it has begun! See you losing weight soon

1.   Get Enough Sleep:

I can't stress this enough, but if you are really serious about losing weight faster,you have to start getting some good sleep.

forget about going to bed late, believe it or not it makes you heavier in the morning right?,

as long as sleeping makes you sweat,AC or not your skin sweats, thereby reducing body mass,and burning out calories without hard work...you see you don't need to work hard to lose some calories do you? ......

Get enough sleep

2.

Don't Sit At A Place For Long:

imagine you are on a boat,and it starts sinking whoooooooooooooooo mmmm

Do you still stay at that same spot you are? Forget about running helter skelter for survival,let's be practical on the side of "Weight" now

I hear you say "no" that's correct! , Staying   at   that   same   spot continuously adds to the ship's weight ,and what will happen,it starts sinking from that side.

But think about it,what if you weren't still sitting or staying at an exact spot ,you will probably be walking around , stabilizing weight,

thereby reducing the risk of sinking from one point and while you walk around,you sweat and lose some calories right?

Okay please do not try this on a sinking ship ,just find a way to get out haha,don't mind me,the most important thing is that you get the logic there,you clearly understand what I am trying to point out.

Now in the case of , damping on an exact spot for hours ,wow that doesn't sound fair , does it? .

You may have realised that sitting on a chair,be it sofa for long , you're getting more heavy literally...

how? You're directing most of your body weight to lump with you,in your stomach,back,and your waist down,and that's not good for you.

Sitting at a place for long brings fatigue,if you're working,get up, take a walk around,grab some water and get refreshed,you will feel much better!

It may just be the reason you are having a bad stressful day at work.....who knows

Think about it ,why do you feel heavier when you stand up from your chair which you have been on for a long time? Well you have directed a lump of your weight down to your belly and waist down.

That's why most "so weighty" people prefer staying at a place,and guess what they can't stand their weight anymore and prefer just damping there.

Walk around.

3.   Taking Light Meals:

Ahhh I see you're shooting nooooooo ,but trust me you have to,just bit by bit,take it slowly,I am not asking you to do like me but sometimes I skip the afternoon meals, sometimes the dinner.

Instead take something lighter,you will be feeling much better,and train yourself and stomach,and reduce its yearning for big foods,it takes determination and focus.

If other people can do it,why can't you? You have already taken the most important step ,I doubt you will be going back now.

This is like a training for your stomach,trust me after some weeks or months,you will be seeing yourself not eating much as before,like I said sometimes now ,I force myself to eat,so I prefer light foods.

You can do it!

4.   Weigh Your Weight Daily Or Weekly:

This is going to be a bit hard,if you don't have the instrument, well if you have access to one ,or a clinic or hospital nearby, but Is a lot simpler now to have a portable one at home,there are many of them.

But if you cannot weigh everyday,no problem,you can still do it weekly!

So,what's the point?

Researchers finds out that when you weigh your weight at least daily or Wednesdays ,you will be in control of your routines and every other thing.

You simply,are going to know what works best for you, the meals that work for you, routines and exercises.

When you weigh your weight try keeping records, either with your phone or on a book,the aim is to keep track and be in control of your routines, watching what gets your weight high or lower,then adjusting with evey result.

Trust me this is an effective strategy,as you don't have to let go of all your beautiful foods,it is now in your hands to choose,not me or someone else to choose for you.

For instance,today is Monday, I have commenced my journey on losing weight, breakfast was tea,lunch was a proteinous food, probably for dinner,I took just fruits and that was it.

Next day, Tuesday,I checked my Weight, recorded it, and tried it once more or something else.

The next day, which is Wednesday,I check my weight,and there might be a slight change,no matter how small it is, wether gone up or down,it is something!

Keep on trying,the purpose of doing it daily is to keep track of your daily activities towards your weight,and taking control of what works best.

In that manner you will get used to it,and if it proves very good for you, stick to it,and before you even realize,you are already adapted to that style which is dope!

If you do it weekly,you may not stick to it, because seeing daily results motivate's you more,but whichever works best for you,it is all recommended!

As long as it all reminds you and motivate's you about the task and commitment you are in,you are good!

The key is keep being motivated!

You can do it!!!

5. Engage In More Activities That Make's You Sweat:

Don't just sit and do nothing,try doing something,it could be anything, remember staying at a place isn't good for you, you can just walk around, walk around till you're tired,or probably done walking.

Help out some oldies do a couple of things,get a skipping rope,skip ,skip and skip,play around with your pets.

Play around with your kids, you can turn to a kid for a moment it doesn't matter anyway, because you will get closer to your children or child,try having some super fun!

Keep doing it as long as you sweat,ride your bicycle,race against friends,do a marathon and more! Play football, basketball, volleyball, anything at at all

You will start seeing changes,not only in your "weight journey" but your life and wellness.

6. Worrying Makes You Lose Weight:

This is not an advice or recommendation,just in case you get into that mood, when mood swings , channel it to something useful and don't let it consume you.

When you're stressed or worried,or anything in that category you get pale isn't it? ,

So, next time instead of letting it consume you,use it proper,and meditate at that particular moment,you will feel much better!!

7. Walk Around Your Home Every Morning:

Just as simple as it sounds, when you wake up,walk around,don't just wake and sit,and then head over to the kitchen to eat.

Not even because you want to lose weight,is not a good style,so if you do it,then check up and change Okay?

Thank you!

You can have your kids do the same.

Just in case you can't run enough,just wake up early enough and do the walking, anywhere you want.

8. Drink Plenty Of Water:

Drink enough water every morning,make it a routine,it also helps you start off your day so well!

You become active and full of energy in the morning and for the day,but it doesn't stop there.

Drink enough water,not only in the morning,but anytime possible.

9. Avoid Taking Heavy Foods:

Avoid taking heavy meals, because it adds very well to your weight,start Making it light,take it lightly and bit by bit.

Don't rush your food also,take slowly, as a king and a queen you are.

10 Replace Dinner "Foods" With Fruits

Remember you are taking it all light as possible as you can.

Hey don't feel bad,it requires a level of Sacrifice,and commitment and a high level of discipline.

And trust me once you start,and keep doing it you will get used to it also.

and when you have achieved your goal,you can go back to taking heavy meals,but lightly and small portions.

You will even get used to taking light foods and eating small,once you have trained your stomach,and disciplined your appetite and yearning for food.

11. Exercise More Often:

Just like a boss in everything, exercise is one of the top boss,in loosing weight.

Whatever you do about it, however you go about it, exercise still remains a recommended routine and a top tip in loosing weight.

Luckily,it doesn't have to be hard,or much stressful,but your energy is required to be honest,it is all determination,you can do it!

You can do simple exercises like, jogging, cycling, swimming, squatting etc.

Boxing is a very good exercise to loose weight fast,I did this when I started mine, spent some good time too,and sweat profusely.

Don't worry we will get to the best exercises.

12 WATCH COMEDIES,JOKES,AND ANYTHING THAT MAKES YOU LAUGH OUT LOUD:

Yes... in this journey you will need this , you need to totally focus on everything that makes you laugh and show your 32 haha I see you're already laughing!

Come on ! Laugh ! Is an essential part of life,we all have to smile at last no matter what,isn't it?

Watch comedies,jokes and more , sometimes you even sweat while laughing, laughing is one of the best medicine in the world!

It really helps, it really does….

<u>**CHAPTER THREE:**</u>

MY STORY:WILL IT INSPIRE YOU? WILL IT MOTIVATE YOU?

This is the question,I would be asking you, you might get everything you want here

tips,exercises, routines,food,does and don'ts, you might all catch everything you are looking for in this chapter.

But the real question still is,

will it motivate you on your own journey?, will you take on the path and act on it?

Will you be determined enough to keep to it? Will you be determined enough to continue your journey no matter how hard the road seems to turn out?

Why not???

You can!! I believe you can,I really do and I know you can!

When I started mine,it was a bit of hard work,but as Time went on and on, I have become used to it all.

And guess what? right now I don't feel like I even did it all,is just like a movie how things changed and it is true, time changes! When you use it Positively.

Now I don't even remember that I had to skip meals at times ,give up on some foods and eat smaller portions of a full plate Upto two to three times! Haha yes I did it,and you too can!!!.

Exercises that worked for me:

Like I told you, you will be going through this with me,this is not just exercises that worked for me, but my recommendable simple exercises that will work for you.

As I said earlier, you don't need to read a bogus page book on weight loss before you can lose weight.

It doesn't even matter how huge and complex it is,the most important thing is , the value of the content.

So I am going to keep it simple and real quick and easy.

You don't have to see loosing weight as some kind of "Wow that's pretty much hard"

Not at all,it should be easier and quick to glance at and grab the information in it.

I started working out about 4 years ago, although it was also for fitness,I was burning out calories very well.

So you are not just going to work for Weight loss,but at the same time working out to be fit!

Here are some best exercises for "quick" result:

Boxing: boxing is one of the best recommended exercises for loosing weight as you really sweat profusely when punching that bag and joggling up and down.

There is no dull moment with boxing,as your whole body moves.

Yes you can go to the gym, straight to that punching bag,take it slowly,try balancing your body ,right to left,left to right before striking.

This is an exercise that ,not only do you lose weight,and get some fats burning,you develop stamina and strength,and a better fit body.

Keep punching it, you can choose to do it lightly, whichever way works,the most important thing is that you're doing it the right way ,and burning off fats.

Have it in mind,if you do not move your body, you are doing more harm than good literally,shake your body,shake it out!

As you can see is like a Duo exercise, you can do this every morning,with your best song being played to your ear.

Dance and shake your body to the music as you do your punching,let it be in your mind that you're doing this for yourself!

For the greater good,I give you two to three weeks and you will already be addicted and used to punching.

 What do you got now? Two things ,you have caught two birds with one stone.

 You will not only loose weight,but keep fit, you will notice Positive changes in your body,just from weeks.

You will still see this,on the best exercises page,just to let you know that it is as simple as you think,so simple! Just a little hardwork and commitment,!

It all takes determination and dedication to it ,it isn't hard work,stick to it.

Yes you can!

I started with boxing:

If you can get it fixed at your home, instead of going to the gym house,then great!

It is also great to have a training partner,so you don't feel alone and bored probably.

I would wake up in the morning, drink enough water and head to the punching bag.

I keep punching it ,while dancing around,is one of the fastest way to loose weight,if not the overall fastest.

Before 30 minutes or so,I have started sweating real fast and heavy,I get soaked,and it is as if I just poured water on myself.

I would jog and juggle left to right,right to left,and punch,balance my weight ,and punch ,just like in a boxing match,how they dance around.

That's mainly to balance their weight and direct it to their opponents with a heavy pinch!

Honestly,it can at a point get intense,don't worry get some rest,don't over stress yourself,don't just do that,you ain't the one who crucified Christ are you? No

You don't deserve to be stressed out,get some rest and get back to it,if you're totally new ,take it easy and slowly.

You will get used to it ,with time.

I do some push ups:
Since I am not training or competing with some kind of world push up champion,I do it to the amount my body can take at that moment.

Push up,was one of my basics,it makes you able to lift your weight.

Do you know that you're weightlifting when you do push ups? You're lifting your own weight,and getting lighter too.

Abs training:
  The purpose of training the abs is to strongly develop a resistance to consuming much.

And no matter how much you eat later,your packs will still be there for you,it is everlasting.

If you will be doing boxing, which I strongly recommend for you to start doing,you will also be building your abs,and other muscles.

You will soon fall deeply in love with your body and you will be like "Wow! Life's Good! " I feel Damn good!! "

That's how I felt too,

Boxing every morning and night ,I started losing much figures,and I was like wow! ,Is just that then I wasn't in love with the figures so I never really cared recording it.

But hey,don't try not recording it,or I will fall out with you,... Understand?

Now we are talking…
So recording it all, motivates you more and keeps you moving!

I skipped meals:

When I feel like,"my packs are coming out Great" I wouldn't want to jeopardize that ,the excitement and joy,at that very moment it brings with eating food,let alone something heavy.

As you train more,and start seeing results, you will be so excited and motivated about it that you wouldn't want to give up,for just a moment of *"food pleasure"* .

As time goes on,you will be seeing Changes in your eating habits and lifestyle.

I did this ,to the point,I only need to take a small quantity of food to get filled up,yes!

It was a bit hard, but I had to,I wouldn't give up running while I was in the middle of the road, would I ?

I get Hungry quite alright, but instead I keep taking something lighter, maybe fruits or drinks,I disciplined myself and my stomach haha…

But know when to just take a break, please this doesn't mean you should keep yourself hungry no, take a substitute, something way more light,than the major meal you Normally take.

Taking small quantity of food:

The main thing is to be determined enough,be disciplined enough to control yourself,your appetite and yearning for a big quantity of food.

Even if you don't eat much ,you know which foods are heavy the most.

So this is how I went about it, normally I would finish up a whole plate which is let's say normal for an average adult.

I cut the food into two,if it is in the morning,I eat the half,and in the afternoon i take the remaining.

Yes it wasn't easy,but I stuck to it,I had it in mind that I am doing this for my better self,and nobody will do it for me,I kept on striving and grinding.

In time,I developed eating a small quantity of food, which is just like normal for me,up till now I still don't consume much.

See,is all about discipline and being determined!

You can do anything! Anything at all!

Yes you can!!!

Giving up some foods, mostly fat and oil

Not your best friend in this journey,is it? I don't think!

So I gave up,on consuming most oil and fats foods,but well sometimes I just take small,to hold my throat haha.

Exactly why I recommend weighing your weight often,to see what best works for you.

Another man's food is another man's poison" that's true here,but to an extent, because there are certain things applicable and working for everyone.

It was becoming visible that I worked out, which the more it gets more visible,the more I worked out.

As simple as it looks,this is what helped me lose so much weight, before going into working out for muscles.

Is simple but requires your commitment to it.

I also went into weight lifting after I must have built myself and so much ready for some Extra work.

If you're going to lift weights take it real easy and slowly, because weight lifting requires food,don't make a mistake.

 My goal was to be light and fit and not to be a muscle man.

You have to know what you really want, before going for anything.

But depending on how "weighty" you are,you can build up your muscles with the fats already in your body by weight lifting and other related activities.

You can do anything you want to do!
Yes you can!

CHAPTER FOUR:

MEAL PLAN(S)

Here are meal plans to go about losing weight, you can still add,and contrast to what favour's and fits you.

But the most important thing is to drop junkies and processed foods, eat more of vegetables and fruits, including whole grains and nuts,foods with low carb at least under 500 cals ,with enough fibre and minerals.

I recommend taking enough nuts at least 4 days a week in the evening, almonds, tigernuts,etc.

Monday:.

Morning: between 6:30am - 7:45am =*Oatmeal*(protein added to every oatmeal breakfast +Veggies)

Afternoon: between 12:38pm(best for lunch) -2:30pm
=Boiled potatoes and Eggs/ (you can replace with any

normal food with a low calorie count with a considerable amount of fibre)

Dinner: anywhere between 6:30pm

=Preferably Pasta with prosciutto , cherry and tomatoes.

Tuesday: inline with Monday's time.

Morning: following the same time and routine,

=*Oatmeal*

Afternoon: whole eggs with vegetables

Dinner:. = Collard sauté with chicken and white beans/ or your preferred meal,but strictly inline with your diet and a light meal always for dinner.

Wednesday:

Morning:. = Oatmeal

Afternoon:.   = Beans/whole grains

Dinner: =Seared salmon salad with BlackBerries.

Thursday:

Morning:.   = Oatmeal

Afternoon:.   Tuna   avocado sandwich

Dinner: Indian shrimp curry

(Check up for the recipe)

Friday:

Morning:.   = Oatmeal

Afternoon:.   = Vegetable sauce
and rice

Dinner:.   = Mixed fruits and nuts.

Saturday:

Morning:.   = Oatmeal

Afternoon:.   = Burger and fries
and enough veggies

Dinner: = Mustard-parmesan
whole roasted cauliflower

Sunday:

Morning:.   = Combined fruits (low Carl)

Afternoon:.   = Rice +veggie and fish.

Dinner:.   = Sautéed Broccoli and Almonds Detox Salad

Now you are probably thinking"What????, Oatmeal every day almost???" Pretty much sounding "not good" don't worry let me land first.

Oatmeal contains a high quantity of fibre and is very low in calories,trust me oatmeal will greatly influence your weight loss journey.

But, keep in mind that this isn't all,you just don't have to go to the grocery store and load up oatmeal no…..

However,the oatmeal you will be taking for breakfast isn't processed already-made ones.

Go for unsweetened normal oatmeal, because most of the company packed Oatmeal may not contain the necessary nutrients you need .

Moreover,your oatmeal shouldn't be just scanty, because with exercise plans , strength training is greatly involved.

And you need a breakfast that can give you enough energy and fill ,till afternoon.

Add Fresh vegetables or natural sweeteners to spice up your oatmeal flavour, raspberries, BlackBerries etc.

Endeavour to add a good source of protein to your breakfast,just not to get fed up with oatmeal Every morning,try different oatmeal Recipes.

You can do it!
The main aim is to combine foods with high fiber supply and protein, consume mostly and more of fruits, veggies, yoghurts,whole grains and

don't forget oranges! Or where you can get a good quantity of vitamin C!

With that out of the way,now is the time to change your junk "snacks" to nuts.

Yes, take nuts in place of snacks,if you can,take almonds or other low calorie nuts high in fibre at least every evening or afternoon,if possible.

All I am saying is add nuts to your plans, however you change it.

However,you don't have to be "restricted" to the afternoon or evening meals , you can take anyone you can make,that is strictly,and I mean strictly low in calories and is a good source of protein,fibre,add veggies to it all.

You can always include green tea, at least once a week.

Don't think it is all,meals and exercises,no,you also have to work more on managing stress and getting adequate sleep.

I can't stress this enough,your body needs it! Your brain needs it!.

And with the exercises you will be doing, you need adequate sleep,and one more thing, keep to about a gap of about 3 hours between dinner and bedtime.

Don't forget, include protein to your oatmeal.

With the meal plans, exercise and the tonic/mix for weight loss, you will lose weight fast enough!

I just give you a month, yes! If it is all good for you and you're seeing good results, keep it up! And know you can also change or repackage your plans.

If you reach your desired goal,you can stop with the ginger/garlic drink and don't overdose.

But absolutely there's nothing to worry about!

Don't over exercise and know when to stop "losing weight".

CHAPTER FIVE:

EXERCISE PLANS:

However you go about it,first things first, you start with strength training and always have a rest at least a day.

So here,you will be resting on Sundays!

Determination is the key!
And to keep on going, you have to;
Judge yourself!

Motivate yourself!

Daily weigh your weight to see what's working best and keeping up on your journey!

Okay for the exercises:

1.)

------ **Strength Training:** (weight Lifting).

= Two Days A Week Monday And Wednesday.

Including, goblets squats,Dumbbell bench press,etc.

Time: 45mins - 1 hour per session

Tips:

...Try to mix up training, at least every three weeks to keep your body more active and responsive to training.

As one type of training might get used to your body,and thus less effective.

Follow each two Weeks with an increased Weight and decreased rest time.

2.)

-------Cardio training steadily:

= Two Days A Week Tuesday And Thursday.

Including Running, swimming, cycling, indoor cycling, skipping rope…

Time: 35Minutes -45minutes by session

Thursday: abs cardio (train your stomach on Thursday's cardio.

3.)

----- High intensity interval training:

=Once a week

Friday…,

Includes: Treadmill interval workout,lower body weight interval , indoor cycling etc.

Recommended: Boxing (your whole muscle and body works,is advisable to have a trainer at the gym show you how to box,so you don't do it the wrong way)

Remember, boxing was my own core, boxing works best for fast weight loss,you shake it all out!

You can do it!!!

Time: 20 minutes per session/or as directed by your trainer).

3 sessions is okay for the day.

4.)

----------Yoga

Once a week

Saturdays

Time: 20 minutes per session for 2 hours a day

5.)

Sundays:

---Rest Rest Rest Rest

And get ready for Monday!

You can ride your bicycle for at least 20-25minutes on Sunday evening.

6. Sleep:

Incase you didn't know,is not just about getting enough sleep,but you can add this to it all

Sleep with two Sleeping bags and four blankets to sweat fats off!

See,is that simple, although it may be uncomfortable for you,but this is

the simplest way to lose body fats
doing absolutely nothing hard!

You will get used to it.

CHAPTER SIX

BEST EXERCISES FOR WEIGHT LOSS:

Swimming

Boxing

Weight lifting

Yoga

Running

Cycling

Abs training

Skipping rope

Russian twist (for abs)

Dumbbell bench press

Conducting

Kettle bell

Indoor cycling

Goblets squat

Barbell back squat

So you choose the best for YOU!!

CHAPTER SEVEN
WEIGHT LOSS AID DRINK:

Now I am going to show you exactly what and how to mix the medicine

What's needed?

Don't worry, maybe your heart was probably pounding rocks haha "whoa is gonna be a hell lot of ingredients needed!can I get it all "

So,this is what is needed, depending on the quantity you want to make,but I'm advising if you just want to test it to see how your body would react to it,then do it in a small quantity, when you're pleased with the results,you will know the quantity of ingredients to mix then!

All you need is
Garlic,
Ginger,
Turmeric,
Lemon
And a diluted alcohol (not beer,but maybe Gin or any form of fresh alcohol that won't harm you)

You can use water to dilute too

The reason (s),for using alcohol is because this solution has proven to be the best ever and works more effectively

How to prepare:

Peel out the garlics,gingers,turmeric and lemon (lime) ,
Don't pound it or anything just cut it all into small sizes, put it together in a bottle or any container and pour in the alcohol, leave for at

least 2 days to properly blend and condensed

Drink a short of it every morning, preferably a tumbler,
Please note: sometimes you have to skip days to avoid excess or overdosage,and have a break when possible.

If you are not okay with alcohol,use water to dilute and let it ferment for 3 days before drinking it.

If you will be using the drink to support your weight loss journey,this is how we will go about it.

You know that these herbal ingredients often have high content of the minerals/properties they have, while some have little or no side effects,you should watch how your body reacts to it and don't abuse it(excessively).

First thing in the morning,(Monday),take a shot of

the mixture, remember to shake it well before use.

Next time to take,will be on Wednesday.

After Wednesday,take on Friday and Saturday,which equals to 4 days a week.

However, you should also note that human body systems aren't the same,your body may be good with 4 days a week,your friend's body may be good with 6 days a week,and just like that.

So if 4 days a week doesn't suit you, you can lower it to 3 days a week or higher.

Not only will you lose weight fast enough,you will see positive changes in your body!

The alcohol solution,works best for flushing out the unwanted bad "stuffs" in your system.

 Great for infection treatment!
Put your alcohol intake to Good use!, but I would advise you,who

wants to lose weight to use water to dilute.

It wouldn't make sense if you're on diet, taking veggies and everything, watching your health and healthy Lifestyle,then taking alcohol? ....well if you can't keep off, reduce your alcohol intake.

Water is Life!

This however isn't a medical advice,and isn't a must and is not a substitute for serious medical attention and emergency,the point here is, embrace nature's foods,they are the best gifts to mankind, taking natural herbs keeps the doctor away.

But garlic,ginger,lemon, turmeric are very good for your body,take it! It gives your body a great immune boost, creating and developing strong resistance to diseases and sicknesses.

Bye to infections,bye to being weak always,bye to diseases and sicknesses that gives you a hard time!

CHAPTER EIGHT

LAUGH PILLS:A MEDICINE FOR WEIGHT LOSS:

Maybe I am the first Fella, maybe not, to ask you to start "laughing" more often , watching more comedies,jokes,and every other thing that's fun enough to keep your heart active , pumping and keep your body sweating!

By the way,it is all about a healthy lifestyle isn't it?

Oh well in case you don't know ,
being happy,and not just "happy"
but widening your mouth enough to
show your 32!

Supports your weight loss
journey,keeps your mind and brain
active,your body losing some
calories,and you being on top of
the world always!

All these factors combined, you are
going to be losing some good
weight in a short while,be happy!

You don't need to look at anyone's face when you're up and laughing like that's the only thing you gotta do!,laugh anyhow you want to,if you like fall anywhere you want to,I got your back for real.

You might ask" what's the use of putting up jokes here" well mister ,miss if you don't have fun,then you ain't living life to the fullest.

Come on! A little fun won't hurt, even if you are serious always just smile a bit…..yeah just a bit……

Hey ...I can still see you being serious,don't fall out with me .....now smile smile smile smile smile!

Yesssss! That's it ,you're great!

Let's move on then,shall we?

Just my little contribution to keep you up!

So, a man someday was complaining to his friends about his

wife being too demanding,this is their conversation:

Man: Hey Joe,you know I am a good man right? And would do anything to keep my wife?

Joe: Yeah man, what's up?

Man:My wife always ask for money,just yesterday she demanded for $300,last two weeks she wanted $150 and this morning she demanded $180

Joe: Whoa man that's crazy, but what does she do with all that money?

Man: I don't know Joe,I never give her any!

James was too obsessed and concerned about his big belly,so he went to see his doctor:

James: Doc,what can I do to flatten my belly? I'm tired of this bump

Doctor: If you want to lose your tummy fat,you should shake your head in different corners repeatedly and stick with it.

James: "Confused" Lol Doc why is that? And how often do I have to do that? ....and the doctor answered...

Doc: Each and every time your friends says "hey Jame boy take some beer"

A woman was ranting about her experience at a friend's party they attended, while complaining to her friend,this is their conversation:

Clur: Could you believe it sussy? I was insulted at that fancy party.

Sussy: what happened? Why?

Clur: the master of ceremony asked me to take off my mask at the party, saying it was scary .

Sussy: oh and you didn't want to remove the mask?? (Concerned)

Clur: (In annoyance) damn it suss I wasn't wearing one!

A boy with his crush,still shooting his shots, finally came up with an idea:

Boy: (In a romantic and courageous tone) : Nina what are the three best words you can say to me that will make me float in the air and be on top?

Nina: yes! Go Hang Yourself!

A fat lady was complaining to her friend….:

Weighty lady: You know,I'm very angry with the talking weighing machine!

Friend: haha why now?

Weighty lady: whenever I step on it ,it says "One at a time please"

"Stacey why are you yelling and screaming so much? Play quietly like Henry,see he doesn't even make a sound"

"Of course not, mother!,is part of the game we are playing,he is Daddy coming back late and I am you,he don't have to make a sound yet"

Following an investigation for an accident scene,some folks were sumouned and were being asked questions concerning the accident ,then to the last man who was really annoyed for being questioned ,shocked the lawyer

Lawyer:"Mr how far were you from the accident scene?

Witness: Thirty-three feet six and a quarter inches back and long.

Lawyer: (taken back) and how could you know the exact figure?

Witness: I Knew ,I knew some fool would ask that question so I measured it.

Battle of the sexes:

tell a man something,it goes in one ear and out in the other.

Man: tell a woman something it goes in both ears and comes out straight through the mouth!

Arguments:

Two men were arguing heatedly about the physical beauty of a Beauty model, nobody was winning the debate,so the other twisted it around to achieve his goal:

"I still think the praises of her beauty are exaggerated"

"Replace her charming eyes,her golden hair ,her seductive lips,her dashing figure and her smooth and slender legs,and what do you have left? " Asked the first man

The other then whispered sadly "my ugly wife"

A lady was called upon to defend herself on a case, about hitting a public transit driver :

Magistrate: woman,why did you hit the poor driver with your walking stick?

Lady: when I got up from my seat to get off the bus,the driver shouted "Room for three more!"

Manager: so,you are here for the job ?
Fool: yes sir
Manager: tell me,do you lie?
Fool: no Sir
Manager:Do you steal and cheat?
Fool: no Sir….

Manager: and do you start work late and end early…..

(just about to finish,the youngman interfered)

Fool: ehmm excuse me Sir, but I can and shall certainly learn all these things Sir"

Jack the village fool: Bobby ya know ,if my brain were offered for sale,it would fetch nothing less than $200,000

Bobby: Yeah,that's not surprising,your brain is worth a big price because it has never been used!

The mistress men:

First obedient husband: when I yawn is the only time I have to open my mouth when my wife is around

Second obedient husband: I bought a book on how to be in control of your own life,but my wife locked it up,and won't let me read it.

Jake has been absent from work for the past two days,the manager was really furious about Jake being absent for such a long time without permission:

Boss:Jake! Ya Good for nothing pig lad,where has your sorry ass been since Monday!?

Jake: mercy good Sire,I have been out helping my countryside sister take care of   her children,her husband has been out of the country and she has 8 children,4 from a different lad,and gave birth to a new born! Making it 9!

Boss: no shit! poor Mrs! she must be a big protective momma bear now!

Jake: yes boss,that's the point,I didn't know you will grab it fast

Boss: You Fool! Grab what now lad?

Jake: you already said it boss,my sister is an animal

Cody after school rushed back home as fast as he could to deliver a message to his parents:

Cody:Dad ! Mom ! Where are you guys???? I need to tell you something important now!?

His parents being curious and eager to hear what their beloved son has to tell them,that made him rush back home unlike before…

Dad: what son? What is it?

Mom: yeah Cody what do you have to tell us? Better be fast I'm in the kitchen

Son: have a seat you two

Parents puzzled and looking at each other,sat down

Son: Dad ,mom, remember when I told you I don't want another brother?

Parents: yes Cody……..and…?

Cody: Well I see you guys are not ready,and won't be doing that !

Parents: haaaa Cody what makes you say that?

Cody: I asked my best friend why he didn't have another brother and he said it is because his parents always have a little balloon in their closet, and since then they never had another child,and I don't see any in your own bedroom closet!

A certain fat man always saw a thin man walking through their street and always wondered why fhe is so thin.

One day he decided to walk up to the fellow:

Fatman: you know you always make me wonder if there was a Famine of biblical attribute where you live .

Thin man: ya know man you make me believe you were the cause of the famine!

Susan, why did you beat up your friend at school ?

Susan: she said I looked like a chimpanzee and hippopotamus joined together 4 months ago

But   it has been a long time she said that,4 months is long enough to forget and forgive…

Susan: yes mom,but I have never seen   a   chimpanzee   and hippopotamus together until today!

Ma Brun: Do you think I can marry my husband's brother when my husband becomes widowed?

Ma pinky tinky: well ,say that depends on whether your husband's brother agrees when your husband becomes widowed.

Uncle: Ok John be a good lad

John : Alright! Uncle I'ma be good for £20 pounds .

Uncle: Huh! That's too much John! When your father was your age he was good for nothing!

Stash: Dad,I've got a stomach ache

Dad: oh son,that's because your stomach is empty ,so it hurts when you haven't eaten.

Stash: really? Now I know why my science teacher always has

headaches,poor man! His head must be empty too….

Two friends visiting a historic museum;

First man: whoa see that big bone,whose bone is it?

Second man: Victor Hugo

First man: oh, I see another bone beside it,why is it smaller?

Second man: probably that's the bone of Victor Hugo when he was a little child.

Psychologist: Mrs what can I do for you?

Mrs: my husband talks in his sleep,what should I do?

Psychologist: give him a chance to talk during the day.

Four little friends were discussing on how their mothers find relief from their headaches:

Pete: My Mother uses a medication on her forehead

Johnny: mine takes some drugs

Cody: mommy goes to the bedroom, probably to sleep

Jackie: my mum only sends me out to play…..!

"Stand still ya old blump! This is a robbery!

"Now hand over your money Or........." threatening the old farmer

"Or what"? The farmer asked.

"Ehmm why? Don't confuse me please,this is my first job"

"Maria if you had $10 and asked your husband for another $10 won't it be complete for your nails?"

"No,I still have only $10 !

Friend: Don't be silly now! you don't know your calculations?

"Hehe but you don't know my husband!.

A husband got a ticket for a show in town, but he thought he should get for his wife,but he remembered the last time he bought two tickets and they ended up running late to the show , when it was almost over,but he loves his wife,so he came up with an Idea

Calling from work:

" Hello Honey I have got two tickets for the movie show across the road

Wife: Aww that's lovely! I will start preparing now

"You better do, the tickets are for tomorrow's show "

Woman: I can always get my husband to my side anytime I want.

Friend: How do you do that?

Woman:I put on bomb shots and makeup and tells him I want to go see my friend, and get some money ! And there he is beside me.

Boy: Why can't I apply for a driving license? I am old enough
Father: very well son,but my car isn't old enough.

A widow,who was remarried,will often nag her second husband,who will always complain.she would ring a bell on how patient and good her first husband was.

Woman to her Second husband: you always complain about my cooking,you ungrateful man,my first husband always ate happily whatever I cook and present to him!"

Second husband: No wonder ,look where he is now!

A simple ordinary country man was hit by a mini truck ,a doctor who was nearby said to all,he was dead.

Upon hearing this he sat up and shouted" damn you! I'm not Dead!"

A scholar who heard his yelling,cried out "lie back down silly man,do you think you know better than the doctor!"

A man who has been separated from his wife for a couple of years,has no money and has nothing to do,

However his two kids were with him and he saw that they may starve to death and the only option for them was to turn to the street to beg for money and food.

The took off, and when they were about to cross the road,a jaguar land rover accidentally hit one of his sons,

The driver came out of his car" oh good God what have I done! Oh I'm so sorry sir I'm so sorry Sir,I will give you $500,000 right away Sir"

The man just there,left in suspense.

The car owner brought out a cheque and gave it to him.

Upon seeing this he was surprised and so happy,that he looked over to the other son

"Son ,you love Daddy right"

"Yes daddy"
"Good! Now I want you to go and lie down on the road so that a car will hit you,I'm getting rich today ,let

me have $100,000,000,you're not
useful to me, this is the only use
you have to me"!

Engineer no-job and a lawyer
An engineer can't find a job so
he opens a clinic and puts a sign
outside
"GET TREATMENT FOR 20k -
IF NOT CURED GET BACK 100k".
A lawyer thinks this is a great
opportunity to earn 100k and goes
to
the clinic...

Lawyer: "I have lost my sense of taste"

Black man: "Nurse, bring medicine from box no.22 and put 3 drops in patient's mouth"

Lawyer: "Ugh..this is salt"

Black man: "Congrats, your sense of

taste is restored. Give me 20k"

The annoyed lawyer goes back after

a few days to recover his money...

Lawyer: "I have lost my memory. I cannot remember anything"

Black man: "Nurse, bring medicine from box no. 22 and put 3 drops in his mouth"

Lawyer (annoyed): "This is kerosene.

You gave this to me last time for restoring my taste"

Black man: "Congrats. You got your

memory back. Give me 20k"

The fuming lawyer pays him, and then comes back a week later determined to get back 100k.

Lawyer: "My eyesight has become very weak"

Black man: "Well, I don't have any medicine for that, so take this 100k"

Lawyer (staring at the cash): "But this is 20k, not 100k"

Black man: "Congrats, your eyesight is restored. Give me 20k"!

13 CRAZY TALKS TO"NVM"

Please hear this..

1. Life is too short to commit suicide Be patient, you'll still die

2. The way I'm so in love with my future wife ehn, I see other girls as my brothers

3. If during sex a woman looks at you straight in the eyes... Slap her!! She wants to get pregnant.
I know these things

4. Just because you're slim doesn't mean you're a Model. Auntie please find something to eat

5. Two days back, I logged in my Instagram after several months.. 30 mins after, I checked my data balance and uninstalled the app. I hate nonsense!!

6. Valentine is the reason most of you
were born in November

7. Dating two short girls is not CHEATING, because half + half is equal to 1

8. Ladies stop forming on social media.. Some of your boyfriends are phone snatchers

9. Anyone who doesn't cheat in a relationship knows nothing about BALANCE DIET.. Trust me.

Don't come and argue with me oo, I'm not feeling well. ....But hey ...don't ever try that!

10. You are short and you'll still be singing "You raised me up so I can stand on mountains"... Sister are you well at all?

11. No matter how rich you are, when you wanna take a passport, you will still pose like the less privilege

12. My pastor always looks at me during offering time since I gave a

testimony that I won a million dollar lotto. He didn't know I only wanted to impress my crush

13. My aim this year was to be madly rich..
I am already mad, it's remaining riches

Hahahahahaha

SECTION THREE:

NATURAL REMEDIES

TO

SOME SELECTED DISEASES

AND

SICKNESS

AND

ACHIEVING

TOTAL HEALTHY AND STRONG

BODY SYSTEM

THROUGH HERBS

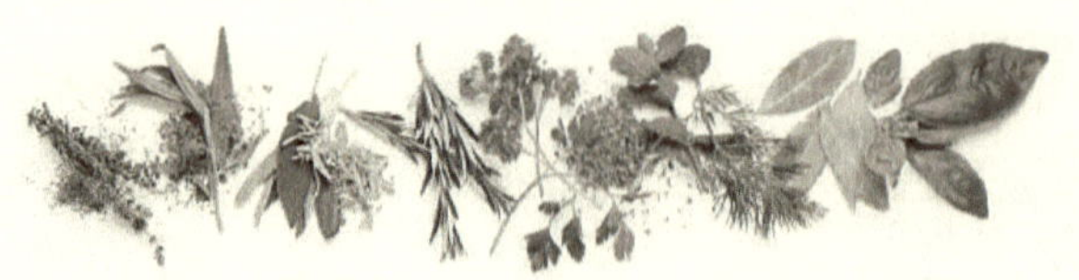

Finally we are in the last section of

this great book!

Welcome!

So hear I would be listing some

sickness and disease you can cure

or prevent

However,these should not be used

as a substitute to serious chronic

diseases or emergencies that

requires professional medical

attention

Bear in mind,most herbs have little

or no side effects,some herbs may

cause slightly undesirable

reactions in "some persons" ,

always try to watch out for any side
effects not only in herbs but also all
other drugs out there,if there are
none, continue the dosage.

INSOMNIA:

Get sorrel juice off the leaves,mixed with castor oil,it is useful for insomnia.

Boil to remove the watery content.

Precaution: the high concentration after boiling is made of oxalic acid, when patients rheumatism and stone in the urinary tract and calculi should not Take it.

CHEST PAIN/HIGH BLOOD PRESSURE:

Get some avocado pear seed,slice and expose the sun or heat to dry for some days,then grind it very well and add 1 tablespoon to prepared Pap ,no sugar Nor milk,take for 14 days .

Chest pain will cease, normal blood pressure will be observed.

Alternative:
Chew garlic 3 times daily.

AMNESIA:

take a pinch of grind Pepper mixed
with honey,take twice daily.

LOW SPERM COUNT/INFERTILITY:

get the leave of cotton, squeeze
with water and add honey ,
preserve in 4 litres to ferment for 1
day

*Dosage: 1 glass ,3 times daily for 1
month*

BLOOD BUILDING:

There are many ways to build up blood, but the most known and healthier way is through herbs , veggies give a lot of aid to blood building
Get many pumpkin leaves, garden egg leaves,lectus, squeeze it all together and drink

It will form a natural hemoglobin
Dosage:1 glass 3 times daily.

HEALTHY NATURAL BABY FOOD:

you will need soya beans,guinea corn seed and millet in equal proportions,grind very well together.

Mix the food,add hot water and sweeten with pure honey

Waist Pain:

10 lime oranges,5 grapes,some ginger,garlic,onions or green leafy onions and add "bitter like" vegetable.

Boil all together in 3 litres of water for 40 Minutes

Dosage: 1 glass daily

Prostate Cancer:

Get some willow herb flower,mix with water and drink a glass 3 times daily till the symptoms are cleared.

Stomach Ulcer:

Have ready about 8 pieces of unripe plantain,slice and grind ,add 4 litres of water.

Leave for 4 days to ferment,shake the content very well in the morning.

Dosage: ½ glass 3 times daily,1 hour before eating, repeat until symptoms stop

Swollen Liver:

Extract ripe mango juice and add honey

Dosage: 3 spoonful 4 times daily.

Sickler:

Take ½ piece of lime orange and a ½ piece of orange , extract out the liquid,mix with an egg yoke together.

Add a spoonful of honey.

Dosage: drink all at once, continue on a daily basis the person will be alright.

Stomach Problem:

Get some bitter leaves and scent leaves, squeeze out the liquid,add water and drink.

When going to bed drink little honey.

PIMPLES/,RASHES/ECZEMA/ RINGWORM/SCABIES ETC:

Get some lime orange,grind some potash add native soap mixed together,scrape the affected part and rub consistently for 3-5 days

Alternative: Get some aloe Vera leaves, grind, with honey .

apply on the affected area.

Acute Dysentry:

Squeeze some quantities of guava leaves with little water,preserve for some time.

Dosage: 1 glass ,3 times daily.

Alternative: get some lime oranges, squeeze out the liquid in a glass cup,add little salt and take.

Should stop it within 15 minutes

Heart Failure:

Take some snails ,remove the inner water (the sticky juice) mix with little salt ,take one tenth of the mixture

Dosage: 2 times daily

Alternative:intake of 100g of onions daily ,assists the functioning of the heart by correcting thrombosis besides reducing blood cholesterol

Minor Paralysis:

take honey with enough garlic mixed together, eat 4 hours daily.

Sore Throat:

take Ginger,add garlic and grind together,mix with aloe Vera Juice and drink

Asthma/cough:

grind two sachets of mustard seed,mix with a 50cl bottle of original honey.
Take 1 tablespoon 3 times daily

Aches(headache/stomach/internal Heat:

just chew some quantity of mustard seed and drink water, enough.

Minor Fibroid:

grind three sachets of mustard seed with black stone,mix with real olive oil or palm oil.

dosage: 2 tablespoons morning and evening ,it will gradually melt out through your "normal waste"

I put "minor fibroid" because this method is more effective to minor fibroid,it may be a little hard for you to find black stone or the Mustard seed,but do ask around,look for natural herb stores ,look up online etc.

Hypertension:

grind 4 sachets of Mustard seeds,mix with one bottle of honey.
Dosage: 2 tablespoons morning and evening daily

Diabetes Mellitus 1:

Take 15 leaves of mango tree,add full cup of water boil and drink daily until it stops.

Worm Expeller:

Some fresh guava leaves,lime oranges and garlic, squeeze together,add little water.

Dosage: 1 glass daily

Nose Bleeding:

use onion juice mixed with honey ,breath into your nose

Memory:

use thyme,boil with water,mix with honey in equal proportions and preserve.

Dosage: 2 spoonfuls into a glass of hot water ,two times daily.

Arthritis/rheumatism:

get some good quantity of ginger and garlic,grind together,mix with 15 pieces of lime oranges ,soak into 1 litre of water , ferment for 1 day

Dosage:½ glass 3 times daily,it will gradually stop x.

Low Sperm Count:

Consume enough carrot or cucumber daily,it gets it thick

Always eat roasted unripe plantain with honey or roasted seeds of groundnut twice a Day

Indigestion/dyspepsia:

Get some aloe Vera leaves,boil with water and take 3 times daily.

It can kill intestinal worm in children ,can be beneficial in cases of indigestion flatulence and constipation.

Alternative:use bitter leave,scent leaves and squeeze together,add some water and add half proportion of honey .
Dosage: ½ glass 3 times daily

Syphilis/toilet Disease:

use lime oranges,garlic,ginger and melon juice,boil together.
Dosage:1 glass 2 times daily

Low Bp:

use some mistletoe leaves,boil and drink after warming in the morning until it stops.

Cataract:

This is a gradual natural cure for cataract,all you have to do is eat unripe strong Banana,fruits, plantain,apple,oranges.

Measles/chicken Pox/small Pox:

Get some bitter leave, squeeze and add both equal proportions if honey and water

Dosage: 3, spoons 3 times daily.

Alternative:take Coca cola morning and evening for 3 days

Pneumonia:

Obtain some quantities of garlic ,pound and mix with 20 lime oranges and 5 grapes , preserve to ferment for 1 day,add ½ bottle of honey.

Dosage:2 spoonful 3 times daily

Diabetes Mellitus 2:

Consumption of 10 fresh grown curry leaves every morning for three months,will prevent/cure diabetes due to obesity and hereditary factors.

It drops the weight .

MALARIA FEVER:

get 25 lime oranges,10 garlics,10 gingers,3 unriped pawpaw,3 unriped pineapple,some lemon grass ,5 grape oranges.

Add 4 litres of water and cut into small sizes allow to boil for about 45-50 Minutes

Dosage;1 glass 3 times daily,must not exceed 3 days.

TB:(tuberculosis):

Helpful:

Eat riped pawpaw seed and main food before meal and ear some garlic before bed ,for 3 days Stop, and continue again until it Stops

Frequent consumption of onions helps.

BREAST CANCER:

grind head of yam bulbs mix with aloe vera and shea butter ,rub on the affected breast area.

alternative;

take your first urine for 14 days and apply the old urine on the affected breast .

TOILET INFECTIONS/SYPHILIS/GONORE HEA/STDs/:

Some tobacco leaves,15 ampicillin capsules,5 wonderful kola pound,add little potash,mix it all with 50cl of hot drink/soda water and about 25 cl of water , ferment for 6 hours

Dosage: shake before use,one shit morning and night for a period of 21 days

IMPOTENCY:

well the cause should be well known before any treatment;

Eating six peppers together with about four almonds daily once with milk ,it is a very good aphrodisiac for the said patient.

Alternative;

Get some pawpaw leaves cooked with water with unriped pawpaw,cut into pieces (cooked together)

Dosage:1 glass 4 times daily.

Stop when you get pregnant.

WEAKNESS OF ERECTION:

Have 3 bug white onions sliced and boiled with water ,filter and mix with enough honey

Dosage;3 tablespoon after meal

Precautions: avoid smoking and alcohol,avoid lime and other Peppered ingridients.

QUICK EJACULATION:

Eat white onion bulbs 3 times daily

SCANTY MENSES:

parsley juice , cucumber juice carrot and beet and squeeze mix with water.

Dosage;1 glass 2 times daily

ULCER:

mix about 50cl of honey with 4 satchets of mustard seed,take 2 tablespoon morning and evening daily.

RASHES IN PRIVY SITE:

Get ½ proportions of scent leaves,some bitter leaves,grind

some garlic and squeeze with little
water
Dosage;½ glass 3 times daily.

TO STOP BLEEDING (CUT,/WOUND):

Use honey and lime oranges mux together dress the bleeding.

These advice are not substitute for a serious illness that requires professional medical attention:
It doesn't matter if you're spiritual or not just hope and pray it works for you!

Be blessed!.

Loads of love .

Please Be Sure To Leave A Positive Review! Thank you!

IG:@CLINTONEMCENT.